HOPE AND HELP FOR

CHRONIC FATIGUE SYNDROME
and FIBROMYALGIA

CHRONIC FATIGUE SYNDROME and FIBROMYALGIA

**Alison C. Bested, MD, FRCP(C)
and Alan C. Logan, ND, FRSH**

with Russell Howe, LLB

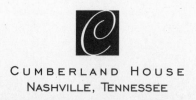

CUMBERLAND HOUSE
NASHVILLE, TENNESSEE

HOPE AND HELP FOR CHRONIC FATIGUE SYNDROME AND FIBROMYALGIA
PUBLISHED BY CUMBERLAND HOUSE PUBLISHING
431 Harding Industrial Drive
Nashville, TN 37211

Cover design: Gore Studio, Inc.

Library of Congress Cataloging-in-Publication Data
Bested, Alison C., 1953–
  Hope and help for chronic fatigue syndrome and fibromyalgia / Alison C.
Bested and Alan C. Logan, with Russell Howe.
      p. cm.
  ISBN-13: 978-1-58182-465-0 (pbk. : alk. paper)
  ISBN-10: 1-58182-465-3 (pbk. : alk. paper)
  1. Chronic fatigue syndrome—Popular works. 2. Fibromyalgia—Popular
works. I. Logan, Alan C., 1967– II. Howe, Russell., 1965– III. Title.
  RB150.F37B48 2006
  616'.0478—dc22

                                                                    2006011643

Printed in the United States of America
1 2 3 4 5 6 7—12 11 10 09 08 07 06

This book is dedicated to all of those brave individuals with chronic fatigue syndrome and fibromyalgia who continue to persist with their difficulties on the long and winding road to recovery, and in memory of Dr. Jeff Sherkey and my dad, Jim Reid, P.Eng.

The purpose of this book is to:

1. Help patients understand chronic fatigue syndrome and/or fibromyalgia.
2. Teach patients tools to promote health and aid in recovery, and help them cope better with their illness.
3. Review current symptomatic treatment protocols, including mainstream and complementary methods.
4. Help patients' families cope and improve the patient-family relationship.
5. Introduce new clinical guidelines for diagnosis.
6. Examine the potential of medications, nutrition, and lifestyle changes.
7. Explore complementary medicine and dietary supplements.
8. Supply patients with information about how to deal with medical-legal problems that may arise if insurance benefits have been stopped.
9. Make people laugh—with special thanks to Jim Unger— because laughter really is the best medicine.

CONTENTS

INTRODUCTION

Patients often ask me how I got interested in the field of chronic fatigue syndrome and fibromyalgia (CFS/FM). As a hematological pathologist, my training included a variety of different fields of medicine, including hematology, immunology, internal medicine, blood banking, genetics, and anatomical pathology. I started my training in anatomical pathology but did an elective training period in lymph node pathology, which turned out to be—for me—a "fascinoma": pathology slang meaning a fascinating area of pathology. As a result, I switched to hematological pathology, which included hematology, immunology, and the other areas listed above. After my training, I spent eight years as the head of a large hematology and blood bank laboratory. I was responsible for the day-to-day hematology and special chemistry testing, bone marrow interpretation, and blood products that were used throughout the hospital, plus the bone bank.

Thirteen years ago I changed my practice. I switched to what I thought was routine outpatient clinical hematology. Things were indeed routine, until one day a patient came to me and said, "I have ME." I said to the woman, "Oh, you have 'me'?" She replied, "No, I have ME, which stands for myalgic encephalomyelitis." I had never heard of ME before, but being a "Mac" grad (my medical school was McMaster University, known for its revolutionary independent learning style) and a pathologist, I said to myself, *I can figure this out*: myalgic—*inflammation of muscles*, encephalomyelitis—*inflammation of the brain and spinal cord*. I still didn't have a clue, so I turned to the "bible" of internal medicine,

Harrison's, to find out something about ME. To my surprise, not a word about ME was mentioned in *Harrison's.* I went back to the patient and told her, much to my embarrassment, that I didn't know a thing about ME, and I asked if she she would mind telling me something about it. She practically jumped out of her chair with excitement and said to me, "You mean you'd be interested?" I said, "Sure, why not?" That one patient was my introduction to ME, which is the British name for chronic fatigue syndrome and the related conditions: fibromyalgia (FM) and multiple chemical sensitivity. Word spread like wildfire among patients, and suddenly I had a practice filled with patients who had CFS and FM (I will refer to them collectively as CFS/FM). I have been interested in this "fascinoma" of medicine ever since.

I was honored and delighted to be selected as one of the members of the Expert Medical Consensus Panel that was asked to write a new clinical definition for CFS. It was a wonderful opportunity to get to know other doctors who are all experts in this field of medicine. The new clinical definition of ME/CFS was recently published in the *Journal of Chronic Fatigue Syndrome.* The purpose of the new clinical definition was to better reflect the criteria and the complexity of all of the symptoms from which patients suffer. It was written with tables and checklists to encourage doctors to work through the complicated symptom complexes that can often be present with CFS.

Having been so ignorant of CFS myself, I certainly understand the difficulty in diagnosing and treating this complex medical illness. It involves multiple systems and presents in various ways. It is a difficult condition to deal with in our current medical system, where there is such a squeeze on physicians' time. As there is no specific delineating laboratory test at the present time, the diagnosis is by excluding all other illnesses that cause fatigue and pain. Once the diagnosis is made, there are general treatments, but no specific treatments suitable for all. The care is generally symptomatic and supportive.

Fibromyalgia can present separately from chronic fatigue syndrome, or it may be present when CFS is initially diagnosed. I learned a great deal about fibromyalgia as I learned about CFS because they are often present together. Many symptoms overlap, and the two conditions have similar approaches to treatment.

This book is intended to provide information for patients with CFS/FM and their families, friends, and doctors. Progress is being made in treating these illnesses; international researchers are working hard to determine their causes and what treatments may or may not be helpful. The authors of this book hope that some of the information included may make your symptoms more bearable and improve the quality of your life.

I was very fortunate to work with Dr. Alan Logan, who spent a year with me while doing his internship at the Canadian College of Naturopathic Medicine in Toronto. Since Alan's graduation (with the honor of being valedictorian of his class), he and I have worked together on a number of CFS research projects. He is a bright, enthusiastic doctor with an insatiable curiosity and a tremendous learning capacity. He has extensive training in complementary modalities with a particular focus on nutritional medicine and is the nutrition editor of the *International Journal of Naturopathic Medicine*. Dr. Logan completed his training in mind-body medicine at Harvard Medical School's Mind-Body Institute in 2001. He has been published in a number of mainstream medical journals, including *Medical Clinics of North America*, *Medical Hypotheses*, *Archives of Dermatology*, and *Arthritis Care and Research*. His most recent article on omega-3 fatty acids and depression in the journal *Lipids in Health and Disease* has received considerable international attention.

Alan convinced me to consider writing a book about my experience in treating patients with CFS/FM. As a result of his encouragement and that of my patients—and a tremendous amount of help from Alan—this book has finally been written. I am thankful to have had him contribute the chapters on nutrition, dietary supplements, and mind-body and complementary medicine. Thank you so much, Alan.

I am very fortunate to have worked for the past three years with Tracey Beaulne, a naturopathic doctor, in an integrative practice. Together in a combined traditional medical and naturopathic medical approach, we have been more effective in treating patients with chronic fatigue syndrome and fibromyalgia. It has been wonderful to see patients benefit firsthand from treatments such as dietary changes, supplements, acupuncture, herbs, and homeopathy. Thanks Tracey, for being part of my team.

The other member of my team, Jack Birnbaum, a psychiatrist, taught me cognitive behavioral therapy. Learning this set of tools has helped me teach emotional energy conservation, otherwise known as stress management, to my patients. I will always be grateful to Jack for this valuable knowledge. Sadly, Jack passed away unexpectedly before the publication of this book.

Russell Howe was introduced to me through a mutual friend many years ago. Some of my patients with CFS/FM were severely disabled and were on the verge of losing or had lost their homes as a result of their insurance benefits being cancelled because chronic fatigue syndrome or fibromyalgia had been diagnosed and submitted on their disability forms. Russ is a lawyer and partner in the law firm of Boland Howe, a small firm in Aurora, Ontario, that restricts its practice to representation of injured and disabled plaintiffs only. Russ is currently the president of the Ontario Trial Lawyers Association and the founder and multi-year chair of the Ontario Trial Lawyers Association's interim disability litigation study group. Russ has spoken at many legal conferences, delivered papers in a number of formats, and published articles on long-term disability and other practice areas in many publications. A significant portion of his practice is made up of long-term disability cases involving people with chronic fatigue syndrome and fibromyalgia, illnesses that Russ has come to understand intimately both through personal experience and intensive study of the medical literature. Russ has also been involved in a number of government committees to effect positive change to the insurance system in Ontario. He continues to lobby and litigate on behalf of disabled individuals in the province of Ontario and across Canada. He has been extremely helpful in educating those within the legal system about this complex area of medicine. Through his diligence, dedication, and hard work, Russ has helped many patients receive the medical insurance benefits that they paid into while they were working. On behalf of the patients who now have a roof over their heads, thank you, Russ.

Thanks also to Dr. Gabriella Chow for her considerable help in writing and organizing chapter eight, which describes some of the pharmaceutical treatments available to CFS/FM patients.

Special thanks also to Ron Pitkin at Cumberland House for publishing this book and allowing us the opportunity to educate, uplift, and encourage those patients, families, and friends affected by chronic fatigue syndrome, fibromyalgia, and multiple chemical sensitivity.

Thank you to all of my teachers from kindergarten to postgraduate school. You inspired me to learn and to continue to learn. When I first graduated from medical school I was like a lot of new grads and thought I knew it all. I have it from the best of authorities that the nurses in teaching hospitals just shudder when the new interns arrive on their floors. I have since eaten my fair share of humble pie and know that I am only beginning to learn. I have had to unlearn many of the "truths" I learned in medical school and learn many new "truths" that are still being discovered. The motto at Kennedy Collegiate Institute, where I attended high school, was *Alteora Peto*—"We seek higher things." I continue to seek higher things, more knowledge, more experience, and more wisdom. I know that as I am seeking, I am achieving. I hope with this book I will inspire and challenge you to learn new ideas. If you have these illnesses, I hope that you will use the new tools presented in this book to improve your individual circumstances and take control of today—wherever life finds you.

Special thanks to my editor, Mary Sanford, who did double duty for this book—you've done a great job, Mary.

Writing a book is a long, complex, and tiring process. This one was written in many places, including in the car and at the ice rink while my kids were at hockey practice. Thanks to my family: my husband, Randy, and my sons, Jonathan and Stephen, for their patience, support, and cups of tea.

God bless you for your interest and for taking the time to read *Hope and Help for Chronic Fatigue Syndrome and Fibromyalgia.*

ALISON CHRISTINE REID BESTED, MD, FRCP(C)

HOPE AND HELP FOR
CHRONIC FATIGUE SYNDROME
and FIBROMYALGIA

CHAPTER ONE

DIAGNOSIS OF CHRONIC FATIGUE AND FIBROMYALGIA

Chronic fatigue syndrome and fibromyalgia have been compared to the Indian fable of the blind men and the elephant. The fable goes like this: The blind men of the village were brought together and shown an elephant. The first man touched a leg and concluded he had hold of a tree. The second man felt the trunk and said that the elephant was a snake. The third man grasped the tail and was sure the elephant was a brush. Each of them described what they had found to one another. Each man claimed he knew the "truth" while thinking that the other men were crazy. A tree, a snake, a brush. How could their ideas be so different? Were they all wrong? Of course not. Each man had a different perspective on the elephant, but no one man had the overall perspective. In the fable the blind men were assuming

HERMAN®

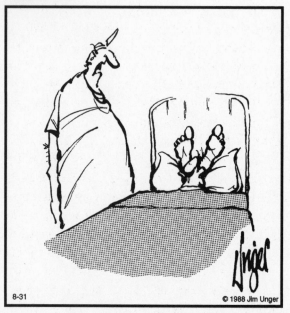

8-31   © 1988 Jim Unger

"It's not as bad as it looks."

that one part of the elephant represented the whole elephant. So in essence, they were all right *and* they were all wrong.

The truth of chronic fatigue syndrome (CFS) and fibromyalgia (FM) is much like the elephant and the blind men. We all have a piece of the puzzle concerning these illnesses, but no one has all the answers. We are still groping.

Over the years, as doctors meet, share their experiences about CFS/ FM, and do more research, the misconceptions about these illnesses have slowly begun to correct themselves. A better understanding of CFS/FM will emerge as the whole picture comes into focus. Here is *my* piece of the puzzle of chronic fatigue syndrome and fibromyalgia.

THE DIAGNOSIS OF CHRONIC FATIGUE SYNDROME AND FIBROMYALGIA

The good news is that you aren't dying. The bad news is it's going to take a lot of time and effort to get better since there is not one specific treatment for CFS/FM. Just how long it will take to get better is not known at this point, because each case is different. The reason there is not a good predictor of the general prognosis of CFS/FM is that researchers grouped patients of different levels of function together, kind of like comparing apples and oranges. New research that takes baseline functionality (i.e., levels of fatigue and function) into consideration is necessary in order to gain an accurate long-term prognosis of both CFS and FM.

I have found that one of the most important factors in prognosis determination is how quickly the diagnosis is made after the illness begins. The earlier the diagnosis is made, the better the prognosis is for long-term recovery. The good news for all CFS/FM patients is that even those who are sick for many years will generally improve slowly over time. However, the degree of recovery is variable. Fortunately, research is ongoing, and we have learned an incredible amount in the past two decades. With the new clinical case definition, earlier diagnosis is now a possibility.

Chronic Fatigue Syndrome

Chronic fatigue syndrome is a complex chronic illness. The following symptoms are usually present: severe disabling fatigue, disturbances in sleep, brain function disturbances (brain fog, poor short-term memory, etc.), muscle and joint pain, difficulties controlling the automatic functions of the body such as blood pressure, stress intolerance, immune system abnormalities leading to recurring infections, and a variety of new drug and chemical sensitivities. Most doctors, upon seeing a patient with CFS/FM come through the door, start to sweat. These conditions bring multiple and complex medical problems. Doctors know that it is difficult to find enough time to truly address these multiple medical problems. Therefore, if you have CFS/FM, I would suggest that you try one of two things: either see your doctor more often and deal with one problem at a time, or, if possible, try booking a longer appointment to address more than one problem at the visit.

Fibromyalgia

Fibromyalgia is similar to chronic fatigue syndrome in that there is a complex set of symptoms that are also poorly understood from a medical standpoint. These include mild to severe widespread body pain, sleep problems, fatigue, stress intolerance, cognitive difficulties, and a variety of new drug and chemical sensitivities. As you can see, there is a considerable overlap of symptoms between CFS and FM, and many patients suffer from both illnesses at the same time.

The problem right now with CFS/FM is that we don't have reliable laboratory tests to diagnose these conditions. Routine tests such as X-rays or laboratory blood work are not yet available to specifically diagnose these conditions. As the cartoon says, "The results of your tests were negative. Get lost." Unfortunately this is all too close to what actually happens when patients with CFS/FM see their doctors initially, because the traditional tests available to help doctors diagnose illnesses have not been helpful for these illnesses. Additionally, CFS/FM as medical conditions

HERMAN®

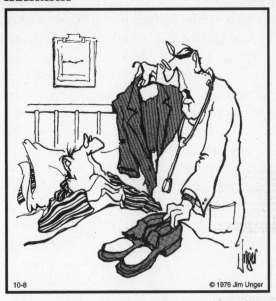

10-8   © 1976 Jim Unger

**"The results of all your tests were negative.
Get lost!"**

have not been taught in medical school because they are newly recognized syndromes validated only by the present generation of doctors. This does not mean that they are new conditions; on the contrary, they have always been with us, but they are only recently described in medical literature.

CHRONIC FATIGUE SYNDROME

Historical Background

Chronic fatigue syndrome is an ancient illness. It was first described in the Egyptian "Ebers Papyrus," circa 1400 B.C. It was thought to have resulted from viral, bacterial, or parasitic infections such as influenza, brucellosis, or yellow fever/infections. Syndromes that resemble CFS/FM have been reported throughout medical literature. Most notably, the diagnosis of neurasthenia was given to patients with CFS/FM symptoms in the late 1800s. Neurasthenia was described as a disease of the nervous system, characterized by physical and/or mental fatigue after exertion, pain, and gastrointestinal disturbances. The severity of symptoms ranged from mild to severe. Certainly sounds like CFS/FM. However, with the rise of psychological therapies, the diagnosis of neurasthenia fell out of favor by the 1930s.

In 1984, there was an outbreak of an unusual flulike illness in Lake Tahoe, Nevada, that began an investigation by a task force from the Centers for Disease Control in the United States. The findings of that investigation led to the first definition and the term chronic fatigue syndrome by Holmes et al. (Table 1). In a number of countries, including the United Kingdom, CFS is often called myalgic encephalomyelitis (ME). *Myo* refers to muscle, and *algic* is inflammation of the muscle. *Encephalo* refers to the brain, *myel* refers to the spinal cord, and *itis* is inflammation. In combination we have the descriptive term that means inflammation of muscle, the brain, and the spinal cord.

In medicine, when we do not have a specific cause for a cluster of symptoms in a patient, we describe the symptoms so that we can look for the new pattern of illness. This is what happens with all newly discovered illnesses. It happened with HIV/AIDS. Initially we did not know what was causing AIDS patients to die. We did know that they all had certain features, including chronic sore throats, viral infections, and immune problems, and that eventually, without treatment, they developed severe disabling fatigue about ten years later and died of unusual cancers (e.g., Kaposi's sarcoma) and infections (fungal infections). I remember as a young pathology resident viewing an autopsy of one of the first AIDS patients to die in Toronto. At the time it was a complete mystery why this very muscular-looking young man in his late twenties died covered with Kaposi's sarcoma on his skin and his organs filled with fungal balls. At that time Kaposi's sarcoma was only seen in very old men and widespread fungal infections were only seen in severely

Table 1. Diagnostic criteria for chronic fatigue syndrome. Holmes et al., *Annals of Internal Medicine* 108, no. 3 (1988): 387–89.

For diagnosis, both major criteria must be present, plus the following minor criteria: (1) at least 6 of 11 symptoms and at least 2 of 3 physical signs or (2) at least 8 of 11 symptoms.

Major criteria 1. New-onset fatigue lasting longer than six months with a 50 percent reduction in activity
2. No other medical or psychiatric conditions that could cause symptoms

Minor criteria

Symptoms (must begin at or after the onset of fatigue)

1. Low-grade fever (99.5°F to 101.5°F)
2. Sore throat
3. Painful cervical or axillary lymphadenopathy
4. Generalized muscle weakness
5. Myalgias (muscle pains)
6. Fatigue lasting twenty-four hours or more after moderate exercise
7. Headaches
8. Migratory arthralgia
9. Sleep disturbance (hypersomnia or insomnia)
10. Neuropsychological complaints (one or more of the following: photophobia, visual scotomas, forgetfulness, irritability, confusion, difficulty concentrating, depression)
11. Acute onset (over a few hours to a few days)

Physical signs (documented by a physician on two occasions, at least one month apart)

1. Low-grade fever
2. Pharyngitis (non-exudative)
3. Cervical or axillary lymphadenopathy

Table 2. Second CFS definition. Fukuda et al., *Annals of Internal Medicine* 121, no. 12 (1994): 953–9.

| 1. **Clinically evaluated, unexplained, persistent, or relapsing chronic fatigue** that is of new or definite onset (has not been lifelong); is not the result of ongoing exertion; is not substantially alleviated by rest; and results in substantial reduction in previous levels of occupational, educational, social, or personal activities; and | 2. **The concurrent occurrence of four or more of the following symptoms,** all of which must have persisted or recurred during six or more consecutive months of illness and must not have predated the fatigue:
• impairment in short-term memory or concentration severe enough to cause substantial reduction in previous levels of occupational, educational, social, or personal activities
• sore throat
• tender cervical or axillary lymph nodes
• muscle pain
• multijoint pain without joint swelling or redness
• headaches of a new type, pattern, or severity
• unrefreshing sleep
• post-exertional malaise lasting more than twenty-four hours |

immune-compromised patients who died as a result of their leukemia or other widespread cancer.

This is where we are with chronic fatigue syndrome and fibromyalgia. We do not know exactly what causes these conditions so we have descriptive criteria to help us make these diagnoses. As we get more information the definitions are updated to reflect this new information.

We do know that these conditions are very common based

on population surveys. A Chicago survey found that 522 per 100,000 women and 291 per 100,000 men were affected. For comparison, breast cancer affects 12 per 100,000 women. The Canadian Community Health Survey (CCHS) 2003 found that in Ontario 0.8 percent of men and 2.1 percent of women who were 20 years old or older had the disease. Women between the ages of 45 and 64 (73 percent of the population of women at that time) had a peak prevalence of 3.3 percent. As you can see, this is a very common illness.

Table 2 highlights the changes in the second definition of CFS. The Holmes (Table 1) and Fukuda (Table 2) definitions are both medical *research* definitions. They help medical researchers to categorize specific patient populations in an effort to identify possible causes and potential treatments for the disease. The research definitions have had their critics over the years. The Holmes criterion was found by the Centers for Disease Control to be ineffective in separating CFS from other forms of unexplained fatigue. The Fukuda criteria have been criticized for being too broad in scope.

Clearly, there was a need for a clear-cut definition for the clinicians who are actually seeing patients in medical practices. Thankfully, an international consensus panel arrived at the new clinical case definition, published in the *Journal of Chronic Fatigue Syndrome* in 2003 and shown in Table 3. The Expert Medical Consensus Panel was composed of treating physicians, teaching faculty, and researchers who had collectively diagnosed or treated a total of twenty thousand CFS patients. I was honored to be a member of the panel.

Exclusions

Certain illnesses must be excluded before the diagnosis of CFS can be made. All of the following diseases have as major symptoms fatigue, sleep disturbances, cognitive disfunction, and pain. A physician must consider and exclude all of them before arriving at a final diagnosis of CFS.

Table 3. Carruthers et al., *Journal of Chronic Fatigue Syndrome* 11, no. 1 (2003): 7–115.

In order to be diagnosed with CFS, a patient must have the following:

1. Fatigue: new onset, unexplained recurrent physical and mental fatigue that significantly alters activity level.
2. Post-Exertional Fatigue: After physical activity there is an increase in symptoms and/or an extended recovery period usually lasting a day or more.
3. Sleep Dysfunction: There is unrefreshed sleep and/or difficulty getting to or maintaining sleep.
4. Pain: There is a significant degree of muscle pain. Pain can also be experienced in the joints and is often widespread and changes location. Often there is a new onset of headaches post-illness. Headaches may be of a different quality and in a different location than in the past.
5. Two or more Neurological/Cognitive Manifestations: confusion; impairment of concentration and short-term memory; disorientation; difficulty with information processing, categorizing, and word retrieval; and perceptual and sensory disturbances. The Expert Panel describes overload phenomena, cognitive and sensory—i.e., heightened sensitivity to lights and noise—and/or emotional overload, which may lead to "crash" periods and/or emotional symptoms.
6. At least one symptom from two of the following categories:
   a. Autonomic Manifestations: blood pressure abnormalities, particularly when rising from lying or seated position, often called delayed postural hypotension; light-headedness; nausea and irritable bowel syndrome; urinary frequency and bladder dysfunction; heart palpitations; shortness of breath with physical activity.
   b. Neuroendocrine Manifestations: "Thermostat" regulation is lost, presenting as lowered body temperature with significant daily fluctuation, sweating episodes, recurrent feelings of feverishness and cold extremities; intolerance of extremes of heat and cold; significant weight change—lack of or abnormal appetite; worsening of symptoms with stress.
   c. Immune Manifestations: Tender lymph nodes; recurrent sore throat; recurrent flulike symptoms; general malaise; new sensitivities to food, medications, and/or chemicals.
7. The illness is chronic and lasts for at least six months in adults, three months in children. It usually has a distinct onset, although it may be gradual.

These exclusions include:

- Addison's disease
- Cushing's syndrome
- hypothyroidism
- hyperthyroidism
- iron deficiency
- iron overload syndrome
- anemias of various types
- diabetes mellitus
- cancer
- treatable sleep disorders
- rheumatological disorders such as rheumatoid arthritis, etc.
- neurological disorders such as multiple sclerosis, Parkinson's disease, myasthenia gravis, B12 deficiency
- infectious diseases such as AIDS, hepatitis, tuberculosis
- Lyme disease
- primary psychiatric disorders and substance abuse.

In my practice I am currently using this new clinical definition to help me diagnose patients with CFS. I find the definition very useful and will go into more details about the criteria of both CFS and FM later in this chapter.

The clinical definition, with detailed treatment recommendations for individual physicians to consider, is contained in the *Journal of Chronic Fatigue Syndrome*, available at www.haworthpress.com; see the Appendix for details.

FIBROMYALGIA

Historical Background

"Muscular rheumatism" was first described by doctors in the 1800s. The symptoms of this condition included pain, stiffness, and disturbed sleep. In 1904, Sir William Gowers, a British neurologist, introduced the term "fibrositis" to describe pain associated with fibrous or connective tissue. In the 1970s, Drs. Hugh

HERMAN®

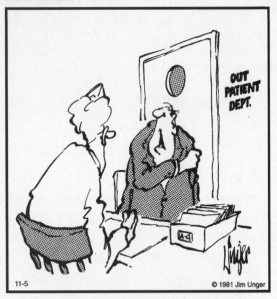

11-5   © 1981 Jim Unger

"Is it OK if I scream with agony between answering the questions?"

Smythe and Harvey Moldofsky found that the symptoms of diffuse muscular pain and fatigue correlated with specific changes on sleep electroencephalograms. The criteria for clinical fibrositis were consequently developed.

The term was changed to "fibromyalgia" and the diagnostic criteria for classifying fibromyalgia were finally established in 1990 by the American College of Rheumatology as a result of a large multicenter study. (See Table 4). The term "fibromyalgia" is a descriptive term. *Fibro* means fibrous tissue, which includes tendons and ligaments, *myo* refers to muscle, and *algia* means pain. FM consists of widespread pain over the entire body that lasts more than three months and has at least eleven of eighteen tender points. If you have fibromyalgia, you will remember the part of the physical examination when the doctor warns you before he examines your muscles that this may hurt when he presses on

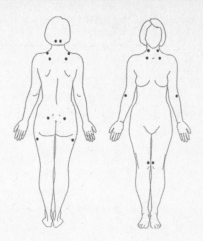

The tender points used to diagnose fibromyalgia.

your muscles—because it *does* hurt when you have fibromyalgia.

More recently, a panel of expert physicians who treat fibromyalgia published a clinical consensus definition to address all of the symptoms that are present in a patient who has FM. This definition is more helpful for clinicians as it gives a more complete set of descriptive symptoms for FM. Fibromyalgia syndrome: Canadian clinical working case definition, diagnostic and treatment protocols—a consensus document, found in the *Journal of Musculoskeletal Pain* 11, no. 4, 2004, includes the original definition in Table 4, and alerts clinicians to key symptoms described in Table 5.

Fibromyalgia affects from 2 to 6 percent of the population, with women representing 90 percent of patients diagnosed between the ages of 20 and 50. Wolfe's 1995 study in the United States found that 3.4 percent of women and 0.5 percent of men had FM. The Ontario (Canada) 2003 CCHS study found that 2.6 percent of women and 0.7 percent of men in people over the age of 20 had FM. Women represented 80 percent of the patients. There is a peak prevalence of 6 percent between the ages of 55 and 60. Again, this is a very common illness.

The diagnosis of FM is often seen with patients who have chronic fatigue syndrome. FM can also be present with other ill-

Table 4. FM definition. Wolfe et al., *Arthritis and Rheumatism* 33, no. 2 (1990).

History of widespread pain has been present for at least three months (pain is considered widespread when all of the following are present).
• Pain in both sides of the body • Pain above and below the waist • Axial skeletal pain (cervical spine, anterior chese, thoracic spine or low back pain). Low back pain is considered lower segment pain.
Pain in eleven of eighteen tender point sites on digital palpitation (pain, on digital palpitation, must be present in at least eleven of the following eighteen tender point locations).
• Occiput (2)—at the suboccipital muscle insertions. • Low cervical (2)—at the anterior aspects of the intertransverse spaces at C5–C7. • Trapezius (2)—at the midpoint of the upper border. • Supraspinatus (2)—at origins, above the scapula spine near the medial border. • Second rib (2)—upper lateral to the second costochondral junction. • Lateral epicondyle (2)—2 cm distal to the epicondyles. • Gluteal (2)—in upper outer quadrants of buttocks in anterior fold of muscle. • Greater trochanter (2)—posterior to the trochanteric prominence. • Knee (2)—at the medial fat pad proximal to the joint line.

Table 5. Additional symptoms of FM. A. Jain et al., Fibromyalgia syndrome: Canadian clinical working case definition, diagnostic and treatment protocols, *Journal of Musculoskeletal Pain* 11, no. 4 (2004).

• Fatigue, particularly post-exertion • Neurological/cognitive complaints • Headaches • Loss of sleep rhythm • Heat/cold intolerance	• Emotional numbness or anxiety • Cardiovascular, dizziness, hypotension, heart rhythm abnormalities • Marked weight change

nesses. Patients can have both chronic fatigue syndrome and fibromyalgia; the overlap between these conditions has been reported at up to 70 percent.

The reason that all of these definitions have been included is to demonstrate that doctors are continuing to grapple with the diagnosis of CFS/FM and that definitions are evolving as new information is available. There are many clinically relevant symptoms that were not included in the previous research definitions. I am sure that if you are a CFS/FM patient reading this book, you can relate to the new clinical definitions which include the reality of a wide variety of symptoms.

MULTIPLE CHEMICAL SENSITIVITY

As outlined in the definition of chronic fatigue syndrome, patients may also develop "new sensitivities to food, medicines, and/or chemicals," which may be classified as multiple chemical sensitivity (MCS).

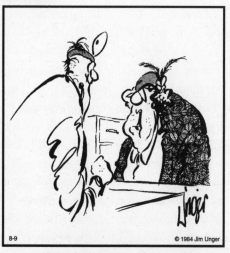

HERMAN®

8-9   © 1984 Jim Unger

**"I feel a lot better since I ran out
of those pills you gave me."**

I was first exposed to the concept of severe food sensitivities while I was a medical student at McMaster University. I remember seeing on a videotape a young man in his late teens being put through the "walk the line" routine that the police used before breathalyzers were available to help them determine whether or not a driver was intoxicated. At first, like any normal teenager, he was able to walk the line with no difficulty. He was given a few drops of beef broth or extract under his tongue and asked again to walk the line a second time. He appeared on the video to be drunk. He was weaving and showing very poor coordination. I was astounded. How could this happen? How could a small amount of beef broth cause such a severe mental or cognitive reaction in this boy? This was my first introduction to the concept of environmental illness and how introducing very low levels of a substance or "chemical" into the patient's body can affect the patient in a profound way. I forgot all about it until years later. But the seed was planted in my unconscious mind.

The production of new man-made chemicals has skyrocketed since World War II, with approximately seventy-five to eighty-five thousand chemicals in circulation in North America by the late 1990s. This number increases by approximately two to three thousand more each year. When individual chemicals (either singly or in various combinations) in household products are released into the air at very low levels, it is largely unknown how these chemicals might affect the health of people at different ages and stages of development (the growing embryo).

In the late 1970s, after a Middle East oil embargo, North Americans were told to seal air leaks in their homes to conserve energy and cut their fuel costs. At the same time, "tight" buildings were built with windows that would not open, again to save the cost of heating or air conditioning the building. The final thing that happened was the ventilation rate (how many air changes occurred per hour) was reduced to save money on heating.

In 1984, the World Health Organization (WHO) reported the following cluster of symptoms occurring "with increased frequency in buildings with indoor climate problems." This collection of symptoms was called "sick building syndrome." The symptoms re-occurred when patients re-entered the same building and disappeared when they were not in the building. (World Health Organization [WHO], 1982, *Indoor Air Pollutants: Exposure and Health Effects Assessment*. Euro-Reports and Studies, no. 78: Working Group Report. Copenhagen: WHO Regional Office. WHO, 1984, *Indoor Air Quality Research*. Euro-Reports and Studies No. 103. Copenhagen: WHO Regional Office for Europe.)

- Irritation of the eyes, nose, and throat
- Dry, red mucous membranes and skin
- Headache
- Upper respiratory infections
- Lower airway symptoms
- Abnormal taste, odor
- General fatigue
- Dizziness
- Nausea

Where I live, in Ontario, Canada, in the mid-1980s, the government created the Ad Hoc Committee on Environmental Hypersensitivity Disorders, chaired by Judge George Thomson, to investigate whether research and clinical efforts were needed in Canada regarding these types of ailments. Their 1985 report stated that environmental hypersensitivity (multiple chemical sensitivity) was a significant problem requiring further research. To assist researchers, they proposed a case definition. They also noted that patients were not getting their needs met in Ontario's health care system. They recommended that patients be treated with compassion and that a special clinic be initiated as a bridge between patients, health professionals, and researchers. As a result, the Ontario Ministry of Health funded an Environmental Sensitivities Hypersensitivity Unit at the University of Toronto in 1994. In 1996, the newly named Environmental Health Clinic opened at Women's College Hospital in Toronto, Ontario. I was asked to join the medical staff at the clinic in 1996 by the clinic director, Dr. Frank Foley, because of my work in the area of chronic fatigue syndrome, which overlaps with multiple chemical sensitivity. As a result of my association with this clinic I have been on the learning curve regarding this illness ever since, along with the other physicians: Lynn Marshall, our current director; Riina Bray; Kathleen Kerr; and John Molot, as well as our clinic staff: nurse education coordinator Gloria Fraser, community outreach coordinator Nancy Bradshaw, and secretary Maggie Messer. Many thanks to all of you for your wide variety of strengths and talents.

In 1987, Cullen reported cases of multiple chemical sensitivity developing in workers after a documented environmental exposure, insult, or illness that could be proven. He proposed a more restrictive research case definition than the ad hoc committee on environmental hypersensitivity disorders (M. Cullen, ed., The worker with multiple chemical sensitivities: an overview, *Occupational Medicine: State of the Art Reviews* 2 [1987]: 655–62). Several other case definitions were published in the 1990s.

In the late 1980s and early 1990s, psychiatrists who had been asked to perform consultations regarding patients linking their symptoms to low-level environmental exposures theorized that ES/MCS was psychological in origin. However, in 1994, Davidoff's critical review of the research literature regarding that theory found little to support it.

Several case definitions for MCS were proposed and published in the '80s and '90s with differing characteristics, but they shared one feature in common: symptoms were linked to low-level exposures of chemicals.

In 1999, a consensus definition was reached on a case definition for MCS by thirty-four North American physicians and scientists and was published in a medical peer-reviewed journal. They found that patients who met the 1999 definition were much more likely to have the following four symptoms: feeling dull or groggy, having difficulty concentrating, feeling "spacey," and having a stronger sense of smell than most people.

Multiple chemical sensitivity, also called environmental hypersensitivity (EH), is sometimes associated with CFS/FM. The symptom overlap is significant, and many CFS/FM patients have a new onset of numerous sensitivities to perfumes, cigarette smoke, diesel fumes, laundry detergent, dryer pads, scented candles, cleaning products, medications, etc. Patients who have MCS can smell odors that the average person cannot detect. The consensus definition of MCS is shown in Table 6.

EH/MCS is a poorly understood area in clinical medicine, and often patients continue to be told that it is "all in their head" or a psychological problem. It is not. It is a physical illness that can be diagnosed once physicians recognize the pattern of the illness. Many illnesses in medicine are diagnosed by pattern recognition; this is just one more pattern to recognize and should be taught in medical schools—as I was taught.

The prevalence in adults is very common. It ranges from 2 to 6 percent in the 1998 New Mexico study by Voorhees and the

Table 6. Environmental hypersensitivity/multiple chemical sensitivity: A 1999 consensus definition.

1. The symptoms are reproducible with (repeated chemical) exposure.
2. The condition is chronic.
3. Low levels of exposure (lower than previously or commonly tolerated) result in manifestations of the syndrome.
4. The symptoms improve or resolve when the incitants are removed.
5. Responses occur to multiple chemically-unrelated substances.
6. Symptoms involve multiple organ systems.

1999 Consensus on Multiple Chemical Sensitivity, *Archives of Environmental Health* 54, no. 3 (May/June 1999); J. R. Nethercott, L. L. Davidoff, B. Curbow, Multiple chemical sensitivities syndrome: Toward a working case definition, *Archives of Environmental Health* 48 (1993):19–26.

1999 California study by Kreutzer. The Ontario 2003 CCHS survey found 1.5 percent of men and 3.5 percent of women are affected. More women were affected, at 72 percent, and there was a peak prevalence of 5.8 percent between the ages of 55 and 60.

IS MAKING THE DIAGNOSIS HELPFUL?

Traditionally most general practitioners or family doctors (about 70 percent) have been reluctant to make the diagnosis of chronic fatigue syndrome. For some doctors it is simply because they don't "buy into" CFS/FM as illnesses. However, the majority of those reluctant to make the diagnosis are fearful that it will only ensure that the patient will live out a life of chronic fatigue/pain. This is referred to as a "self-fulfilling prophecy." However, in reality the diagnosis of CFS/FM has been shown to be very helpful for patients. If the patient fits the diagnosis, it needs to be made. Individuals who live in the dark, not knowing what they have, are clearly worse off. Only through a diagnosis can recovery begin. Research supports this, as almost 90 percent of patients believe that their diagnosis was the most helpful factor in managing their symptoms.

EXPLANATION OF THE CFS/FM CRITERIA

Fatigue

Fatigue is a very difficult word to define. What may be fatiguing to one person may not be a problem for another. In terms of illness, fatigue is best understood if it's looked at in terms of activity levels. The fatigue of CFS/FM is abnormal. There is a loss of physical, mental, and emotional stamina leading to a substantial reduction in the patient's activity level compared to when they were well. The body is very slow to recover and often takes more than twenty-four hours for full recovery after exertion. This is the post-exertional part of the fatigue. For example, if a person with CFS/FM goes grocery shopping for thirty minutes, she may be in bed for a whole day—or maybe even a few days—afterward. In addition, the other associated symptoms of the illness also worsen. There is also mental fatigue, which patients often describe as "brain fog." This may occur after reading, trying to pay bills, or any mental exertion. It may also occur after being overloaded by sound or noise, such as after attending a birthday party or other social event. Fatigue also occurs after emotional events: having a fight with your kids or attending a funeral. Any time energy of any kind has been spent, fatigue can occur.

Sleep Dysfunction
Most patients suffer from sleep disturbance. For some CFS/FM patients it is difficult to either *get* to sleep or *stay* asleep. For almost all patients, after the onset of illness, no matter how much sleep they get, even twelve to fourteen hours, it never seems to be enough. Patients crave a night of sleep that can actually make them feel refreshed or restored in the morning.

Pain
Most patients have pain in their joints (arthralgia) and muscles (myalgia) without any noticeable redness or swelling. The severity may vary from day to day, even hour to hour. In addition, the pain may migrate to and from a number of locations. Often they have significant headaches that differ in location or severity as compared to headaches they experienced before they had CFS/FM.

Most people diagnosed with FM say that they ache or have pain all over their bodies. The type of pain varies and may be described as burning, aching, shooting, stabbing, or tingling. In some people, the pain can be intense enough to interfere with daily tasks, and uncontrolled pain symptoms plus severe fatigue may lead to difficulty sustaining employment.

Brain Function Disturbances (Neurocognitive Dysfunction)
CFS/FM patients suffer from "brain fog." Brain fog is the term patients use when they have difficulty with concentration, short-term memory, word retrieval, and slowed mental processing.

Patients often suffer from feeling overloaded or overstimulated, not only physically but also mentally and emotionally. For example, patients find that attending a social gathering with many people can be extremely draining. They do not have the energy required to screen out background noises or conversations and concentrate specifically on the person they are speaking with. There may also be emotional lability, that is, emotional highs and lows. Anxiety or panic attacks often occur. Reactive depression as a result of being chronically ill may also develop.

Automatic Body Function Disturbances (Autonomic, Neuroendocrine, and Immune Dysfunction)

In general terms, this is the body's inability to maintain *homeostasis*, or normality, in the automatically controlled systems in the body. These systems include controlling blood pressure, temperature, and the immune system. One autonomic symptom is orthostatic hypotension—dizziness or lightheadedness after standing up from a prone or a sitting position. Fatigue is often part of this feeling. Arrhythmias, or irregular heart rhythm, may be present. There may be shortness of breath with exertion. Patients may feel very cold and at other times be sensitive to heat, because the body's temperature regulating system is not functioning normally. They may have episodes of feeling flushed and sweaty even at room temperature. This may happen at night and present as "night sweats."

Intestinal irregularities may be present, which may include anorexia or the opposite abnormal increase in appetite, nausea, or marked weight gain or loss. Symptoms of irritable bowel syndrome may be present with cramping pain, bloating, and alternating diarrhea and constipation. Irritable bladder with urgency and frequency of urination may also be found.

Immune Symptoms

Patients often have sore throats, tender glands (lymph nodes), flulike symptoms, and general malaise (vague feeling of illness). These symptoms can come and go and are often present at the beginning of the illness. Allergies may appear, and new sensitivities to food, drugs, and chemicals can often present, even in the absence of an allergic history.

Length of Illness Requirements

There are some differences in the time frame for the diagnosis of CFS and FM. For CFS, usually the symptoms begin suddenly and persist for longer than six months. In children, the diagnosis can be made after three months. In some people, the onset of illness is more gradual. In the case of FM, the widespread pain must persist for at least three months for a diagnosis to be made. MCS has no time frame attached to its diagnosis.

As shown in the graphs below and on the next page, a study of 134 CFS patient questionnaires that were reviewed by Dr. Logan showed that most cases of CFS that have a sudden onset occur during the Northern Hemisphere flu season, which occurs yearly from September to March.

SOME STATISTICS TO CONSIDER

- 25 percent of all patients in a general practice report fatigue as a symptom.
- 10 to 12 percent of the general population report chronic widespread pain.
- CFS is present in 522 women per 100,000 and 291 men per 100,000.

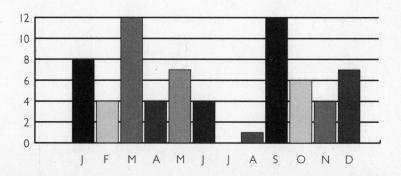

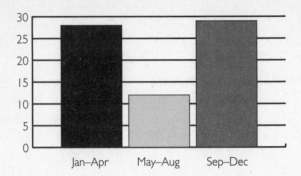

- FM is present in 3,400 women per 100,000 and 500 men per 100,000.
- AIDS is present in 12 women per 100,000.
- Breast cancer is present in 26 per 100,000.
- Diabetes is present in 900 women per 100,000.
- Heart disease is present in 3,400 women per 100,000.
- Arthritis is present in 3,800 women per 100,000.

Reference: L. A. Jason et al., *Archives in Internal Medicine* 159 (Oct 1999): 2129–37.

REFERENCES

National Library of Medicine

By using a MEDLINE search, a comprehensive list of references for CFS/FM can be obtained. MEDLINE accesses the official online archives of the National Library of Medicine in the United States. This Web site is freely accessible by all users. Go to http://www.ncbi.nlm.nih.gov/entrez/query.fcgi?db=PubMed, the online home of MEDLINE. In the "search for" box enter FATIGUE SYNDROME, CHRONIC and click the "go" button. For fibromyalgia information, enter FIBROMYALGIA and click "go."

Centers for Disease Control (CDC) and Prevention

The CDC provides considerable information about CFS on their Web site. Go to their CFS home page at http://www.cdc.gov/ncidod/diseases/cfs/index.htm

How are CFS/FM and Depression Different?

- Desire and motivation to be active remains more pronounced in CFS/FM. Depressed patients lose their motivation and can't get going.

- Intensity of pain/fatigue is usually higher in CFS/FM.

- Sudden onset is more common in CFS/FM.

- More severe neurocognitive deficits are seen in CFS/FM.

- Hypersensitivities and numerous bodily symptoms, while present in depression, are more common to CFS/FM.

- The level of exercise that can improve the mood in depression may worsen CFS/FM symptoms.

References for MCS

References for multiple chemical sensitivity can be found at the Web site at Women's College Hospital site of Sunny-brook and Women's College Health Sciences Centre at http://www.womenshealthmatters.ca. Under the title *Women's Health Matters*, click Enter, then in the topic list on the lefthand side of the page, click Health Centres, then Environmental Health. CFS, FM, and MCS are all present. Another helpful site is www.mcs-global.org

CHAPTER TWO

INVESTIGATIONS AND THEORIES OF ILLNESS

This chapter will explore the current investigations for CFS/FM and will review the theoretical causes of these conditions. It will also touch on future areas of research in these areas.

BLOOD TESTS

The typical screening blood work for CFS/FM is often not revealing or negative. The tests are done to exclude all other treatable causes of chronic fatigue as listed in the exclusion of active disease in the new 2003 clinical definition by Carruthers et al. (see chapter 1). These tests are as follows:

- Complete Blood Count (CBC)
- Erythrocyte Sedimentation Rate (ESR)
- Serum electrolytes
- Glucose
- Calcium
- Red blood cell magnesium
- Phosphorous
- Thyroid stimulating hormone
- Protein electrophoresis screen
- C-reactive protein (CRP)
- Ferritin
- Creatinine
- Rheumatoid factor
- Antinuclear antibody
- Creatinine phosphokinase (CPK)
- Liver function tests (GGT, AST, ALT)
- Urinalysis

Additional tests are done depending on the patient's history, and screening for hepatitis B and C, tuberculosis, and HIV is done routinely, as they are all potentially treatable illnesses.

Because I have a special interest in this field, many of my patients' blood samples are tested using flow cytometry testing. This is a very sophisticated testing method that analyzes the lymphocyte subsets in the blood—similar to the testing done on AIDS patients. This testing often shows decreased T suppressor lymphocyte subsets and decreased natural killer cells. This shows a shift in the immune system and is commonly seen in patients with CFS. In the United States measurement of natural killer cell activity is also available. This activity is often decreased. What this means is that the surveillance arm of the body's immune system is functioning below normal. It is interesting to note that I have not seen an increase in cancers in this patient population so far. But it also means that if you have CFS and you have a history of cancer in your family you must make sure that you are properly screened on an ongoing basis to try to detect a cancer early and get treatment early, because we just don't know if there is an increased risk if you have CFS/FM.

BRAIN IMAGING

We can be thankful that modern brain imaging techniques can look under the skull to uncover even subtle abnormalities in the brains of those with CFS/FM. Exciting new studies using modern brain imaging validate these illnesses. This research shows differences in the nervous system of CFS/FM patients versus patients with other illnesses and healthy controls. The studies are relatively small, and certainly larger brain imaging studies still need to be done. However, the results show that CFS/FM actually *is* "in the patient's head"! Here are some of the findings.

- Decreased blood flow to some areas of the brain on the brain SPECT scan.
- Decreased glucose uptake by certain areas of the brain.
- Small lesions in various areas of the brain on the MRI scan. These are known as "white matter abnormalities," and are also observed in multiple sclerosis. The CFS patients with MRI brain abnormalities reported being more physically impaired than those without brain abnormalities on the MRI scan. (D. B. Cook et al., Relationship of brain MRI

abnormalities and physical functional status in chronic fatigue syndrome, *International Journal of Neuroscience* 107 [March 2001]: 1–6.)

- Reduction in global gray matter volume on the MRI scan in CFS patients compared to controls. This decrease in volume was linked to the reduction in physical activity. (F. P. de Lange et al., Gray matter volume reduction in the chronic fatigue syndrome, *Neuroimage* 26 [July 2005]: 777–81.)

- Enhanced turnover of important phospholipids that surround the brain cells. This indicates a breakdown in nerve cells and can account for the findings of enlarged ventricles. Some researchers have proposed, and at least one published case report shows via MRI, that fish oil high in eicosapentaenoic acid (EPA) can reverse this breakdown. One gram of EPA daily led to a reduction in ventricular volume in a CFS patient assessed with MRI. EPA is further discussed by Dr. Logan in chapter 5.

- The presence of MRI abnormalities in CFS is related to a decrease in functional status. Functional MRI studies showed that CFS patients who have difficulties with complex auditory processing have to exert greater effort to process auditory information on functional MRIs compared to healthy controls. (G. Lange et al., Objective evidence of cognitive complaints in Chronic Fatigue Syndrome: an fMRI study of verbal working memory, *Neuroimage* 26 [June 2005]: 513–24.)

- Abnormalities in pain processing areas of the brain have been documented in FM via functional MRI scans. The results suggest a biological mechanism contributing to the increased sensitivity to pain in FM.

PAIN IN FIBROMYALGIA

A brain-scan study using functional magnetic resonance imaging (f[MRI]) performed in Ann Arbor, Michigan, confirmed that fibromyalgia patients experience pain at a higher degree than healthy adults.

In fact, the study found, people with fibromyalgia say they feel severe pain and have measurable pain signals in their brains from a gentle finger squeeze that barely feels unpleasant to people without the disease. The squeeze's force must be doubled to cause healthy people to feel the same level of pain—and their pain signals show up in different brain areas. (R. Gracely et al., *Arthritis and Rheumatism* 46, no. 5 [May 2002].)

This study offers the first objective method for corroborating what fibromyalgia patients report they feel and what's going on in their brains at the precise moment they feel it. It gives researchers a road map of the areas of the brain that are most—and least—active when patients feel pain. The reason for the neuroamplification of the pain signals was unknown in FM.

SLEEP STUDIES

CFS/FM patients often report sleep-related problems, including difficulty falling asleep and staying asleep and getting fewer hours of sleep overall. Most patients report that their sleep quality is poor and that they never truly feel as if they are in deep sleep. There are objective findings to substantiate this. CFS/FM patients have been the subject of laboratory sleep studies. Disordered sleep physiology is present. This includes abnormalities in brain waves (alpha rhythms) with multiple sleep interruptions during the sleep cycles. The sleep studies often show reduced stage 3 and 4 sleep down to zero. This means that the patient gets no restorative sleep. No wonder patients wake up tired all the time. Indeed, the sleep disturbances of CFS/FM are of a different quality/structure than that observed in multiple sclerosis and otherwise healthy adults.

Sleep apnea, or the condition in which a patient stops breathing momentarily while sleeping, usually results in low sleep quality because the patient wakes up, disturbing the sleep cycle, whenever they stop breathing. If you have sleep apnea, it should be actively treated with a CPAP (Continuous Positive Airway Pressure) machine at night. It is a struggle to get used to these machines, and it may take many different masks and setting adjustments before a patient feels comfortable, but it is worth the struggle, because it will remove one layer of fatigue if the sleep apnea is treated. However, curing sleep apnea does not cure CFS/FM. Many of my patients were told this by well-meaning sleep doctors who did not realize that they also had CFS/FM.

This is where the sleep hygiene routine and the use of sleep-inducing herbs and medicines are helpful (see chapter 3).

NEUROENDOCRINE DISTURBANCES

In order to effectively deal with stress, humans must have the hypothalamic-pituitary-adrenal (HPA) axis working in optimal fashion. Although the neurophysiology behind the HPA axis is complex, at a fundamental level it is quite straightforward. It goes like this: Stress causes the hypothalamus in the brain to secrete Corticotropin Releasing Hormone, or CRH; this in turn causes the small pituitary gland in the brain to secrete Adrenocorticotropic Hormone, or ACTH. This hormone or chemical signal is released into the blood and arrives at the adrenal glands, which are stimulated to secrete cortisol. The secretion of cortisol is essential in dealing with *acute* stress and is normally turned off when the stressor is dealt with by a negative feedback loop.

In patients with CFS/FM, this process seems to be exhausted or, as described in the medical literature, "blunted." Most, but not all, studies have shown that CFS/FM patients have low levels of cortisol, and the cause may be at the top of the HPA axis. It seems that the hypothalamus in brains of CFS/FM patients does not secrete enough CRH, so ACTH doesn't stimulate the adrenal glands and cortisol levels are, in turn, low or on the low end of the "normal" range. The reason for this disturbance is unclear, but one theory is an overused stress response and dominance of the sympathetic (fight or flight) branch of the nervous system over the parasympathetic nervous system, which helps the body to relax. The end result is exhaustion of the system, primarily at the brain level. If the brain doesn't appropriately (i.e., only when needed) stimulate the adrenal glands to secrete cortisol, the adrenals will presume they are no longer required and shrink. This is exactly what has been observed in one small CFS study— adrenal glands that are 50 percent smaller than those with depression and healthy controls. This could explain the intolerance to stress in CFS/FM. The evidence of under-functioning of the adrenal glands may also contribute to chemical and environmental sensitivities seen in CFS/FM patients.

So if in your pre-illness life you were described as a Type A personality and an "adrenaline junkie" and you thrived on stress and the euphoria associated with trying to meet deadlines at the last minute, things have dramatically changed for you. You can no longer "push" yourself because your adrenal glands, the source of your "fix," are now tapped out or depleted. This is the reason you need to learn to pace yourself—because you have no adrenal reserve to help you push yourself to accomplish the long list of the things you want to do. (See chapter 3.)

AUTONOMIC AND CARDIAC MANIFESTATIONS

Patients often complain of dizziness upon standing (postural hypotension) and cardiac arrhythmia (irregular heartbeat or palpitations). When they stand up quickly, they feel like they are going to faint. It has been documented that CFS patients are worse off on the tilt-table test, using the methodology that was specifically designed to test CFS patients. It can provoke low blood pressure, fainting, and many of the symptoms of the illness. One of the major contributors here may be the low blood volume observed in CFS. I often ask patients to increase their salt intake if they have these symptoms and their blood pressure is low. Adequate intake of salt and water is crucial in maintenance of normal blood volume in CFS. The other contributing factor may be a lack of heart rate variability in CFS. The ability of the heart to respond to postural

STRESS ⟶ BRAIN ⟵ STRESS

CRH ↓

ACTH ↓

In CFS/FM this system is
malfunctioning at the brain level.

Adrenal Glands ⟵

Cortisol ↓

In CFS/FM the adrenals
become exhausted.

changes or changes in body position from sitting to standing, for example, and to stress allows control of blood flow to the brain and vital organs. CFS/FM patients appear to have compromised heart rate variability. The feedback loop from the brain to the heart does not seem to work effectively in many patients.

New research indicates that some CFS patients have abnormal cardiac wall motion, which means that the pumping action of the heart is disturbed. This can account for some CFS symptoms, because blood flow and heart rhythm can be affected. The researchers suggest that the abnormal cardiac wall motion is virally induced and is known as cardiomyopathy, or inflammation of the heart muscle. Findings are in line with other observations in CFS/FM, such as reduced blood flow from the heart, reduced circulation to exercising muscles, and/or a post-exercise reduction in brain blood flow.

NEUROPSYCHOLOGICAL TESTING

Most CFS/FM patients report cognitive impairment ranging from minor to severe. It may or may not be consistent, and it varies in intensity from time to time. Physical exertion may worsen the

Using abdominal imaging (CT scans) researchers found the following:

- The adrenal glands of CFS patients were more than 50 percent smaller than those of fifty-five healthy subjects measured. The release of cortisol, a key hormone in stress responses, is lower in CFS patients.
- This is thought to be due to the reduced stimulation from the governing area of the brain called the pituitary gland.
- The low threshold or intolerance to stress reported by CFS/FM patients is very likely a result of adrenal shrinkage (atrophy) and low cortisol levels.

cognitive difficulties. Those with FM refer to it as "fibro-fog." CFS patients often call it "brain fog." The most common complaints are poor concentration, decreased memory for recent events, and decreased recognition of words. Research, by way of standardized neuropsychological tests, has confirmed the presence of subtle and/or significant deficits in cognitive function. Slowed processing speed, impaired working memory, inability to multitask, and poor learning of information are the most significant features of CFS/FM. Indeed, researchers have concluded that the evidence does not suggest that the cognitive difficulties are solely attributable to fatigue, anxiety, or depression. In fact CFS/FM patients are usually highly motivated, as seen by their tendency to push themselves and to do too much on their good days. This is the opposite of depressed patients, who cannot motivate themselves to get moving and are often inert. This is also distinguishable from somatization disorder, which is excluded when the criteria for CFS/FM are met.

For CFS/FM patients this is good news. You do not have Alzheimer's disease. Imagine that our brain is like a filing cabinet full of files. Normally your files are in alphabetical order, and when you want to remember a subject you quickly reach in and grab the correct file and use it. This represents your ability to remember and process information quickly. With CFS/FM, you still have that filing cabinet, meaning that your IQ is still essentially the same. However, the inside of your filing cabinet looks like someone has gone in, pulled all of the files out, mixed them all up, and then shoved the files back any old way. As a result, it takes you time to sort through the files to even *find* the right file (hence your slowed processing and your groping for words). The good news is that you *can* put your files back in order; your brain has the capacity to learn because it has new baby or stem cells that you can teach how to function. You can strengthen your mental processing skills by relearning old materials you used to know, such as your math times tables, addition and subtraction, and language skills such as words, spelling, and grammar. It takes a great deal of practice and use of all the different ways of learning: visual (seeing), auditory (listening), and kinesthetic (writing). How do you get to Carnegie Hall? Practice, practice, practice.

METABOLISM

Abnormalities in the muscles of CFS/FM patients have been documented. In particular, patients have abnormalities within the mitochondria, the important energy pack (or battery) of cells. Patients may not be producing enough ATP, which is one of the energy molecules of life, within muscle cells. When most healthy people exercise for extended periods, they notice fatigue and cramping when shifting into anaerobic metabolism. In the anaerobic state, lactate is produced. Patients with CFS/FM may have an early shift into anaerobic metabolism, with accelerated glycolysis and increased production of lactic acid. As a result, they have an abnormal exercise response and exacerbation of their symptoms after exercise.

GENETICS

ME/CFS

CFS patients were found to have fifteen up-regulated genes and one down-regulated gene. This profile suggested T-cell activation, disturbance of neuronal and mitochondrial function, links with organophosphate exposure, and virus infection. (N. Kaushik et al., Gene expression in peripheral blood mononuclear cells from patients with chronic fatigue syndrome, *Journal of Clinical Pathology* 58 [2005]: 826–32.)

Another article showed differences in cellular ion transport and ion channel activity at rest in ME/CFS cases and controls, exaggerated after exercise with different expression of exercise-responsive genes. (T. Whistler et al., Exercise responsive genes measured in peripheral blood of women with chronic fatigue syndrome and matched control subjects, *BMC Physiology* 5, no. 1 [March 24, 2005]: 5.)

Fibromyalgia

Genetic studies are ongoing. One study showed the presence of COMT gene polymorphisms. It is postulated that this may predispose to FM and be pathogenetically involved through adrenergic mechanisms. This may affect ability to inactivate catecholamines and catecholamine-containing drugs contributing to the pain of fibromyalgia. (S. Gursoy et al., Significance of catechol-O-methyltransferase polymorphism in fibromyalgia syndome, *Rheumatology International* 23, no. 3 [May 2003].)

Multiple Chemical Sensitivity

Drs. Gail Eyssen and Lynn Marshall and colleagues from the University of Toronto have discovered possible genetically related differences in the way those patients with chemical sensitivities deal with toxins in the liver. The cytochrome P450 enzymes in the liver are responsible for handling both external toxins and internal toxins produced by the body. Steady activity of these enzymes is critical; they can't operate too slowly or too quickly in detoxification. The study showed that patients with multiple chemical sensitivity were "different from the controls in genetic polymorphisms in drug-metabolizing enzymes." (G. McKeown-Eyssen et al., Case control study of genotypes in multiple chemical sensitivity: CYP2D6, NAT1, NAT2, PON1,

PON2, MTHFR, *International Journal of Epidemiology* 33 [2004]: 1–8.)

Immune Abnormalities

A study published in *Lancet* validates the symptoms of those patients with food intolerance and demonstrates a physiological mechanism for food intolerances and challenged the false assumption that food intolerances are caused by a psychiatric disorder. In the study, by Jacobsen et al. (2000), patients with perceived food intolerance were asked to consume foods they had previously eliminated. The patients had normal routine laboratory tests and no lactase deficiency. After consuming the milk and wheat for two weeks, those with food intolerance were found to have significant elevations in certain cytokines (chemicals that moderate immune and inflammatory responses). The increase in the cytokines, according to the researchers, accompanied and accounted for increases in abdominal discomfort, headache, and joint and muscle pain—symptoms that are obviously similar to those observed in CFS patients.

As previously mentioned, the role of infectious agents in both CFS and FM onset has been investigated. While post-infectious associations have been made (particularly with CFS), there is no singular viral, bacterial, or microbiological agent that causes CFS/FM. Although some investigators continue to pursue these avenues, most researchers have turned their attention elsewhere.

New research suggests that it may not be so much the infectious agent that started the process but rather the fallout afterward. Immune abnormalities have been documented in CFS/FM, again mostly CFS, as the bulk of the research is here. Elevation of cytokines may play a role in contributing to CFS/FM symptoms. Cytokine elevation can account for pain, fatigue, cognitive difficulties, anxiety, and depression.

The immune status of CFS/FM patients is complex; some aspects appear to be suppressed (cellular immunity), while other areas (humoral [antibody] mediated immunity) in the immune system are activated in CFS/FM. Natural killer cells—important cells that protect against viruses, intracellular bacteria, and cancer—appear to be low in CFS but not in FM. In the case of CFS, a new theory suggests that the initial infection (virus) leads to the usual antiviral response; however, this antiviral response is never properly shut down. Interestingly, this disturbance of the viral defense system (Rnase L) does not appear to be present in patients who only have FM.

In CFS it is postulated that failure to shut down the Rnase L viral defense system leads to a disturbance in this system with an abnormal Rnase L being produced. This results in damage to tiny channels that regulate cellular function in the cell's membrane. This can have a variety of consequences and can account for the numerous symptoms that may present in CFS. For example, if channel "X" is disrupted in the brain, there would be increased sensitivity to toxic chemicals. If channel "Y" is disrupted, there would be increased pain felt in the muscles. If channel "Z" is disrupted, there would be potassium losses from inside the cell and metabolism would be altered with increased fatigue. The fact that channels are present on all cells throughout the body could potentially account for the myriad of signs and symptoms present at the same time in these patients and could explain the multiple symptom complexes that are seen. (K. De Meirleir, *Chronic Fatigue Syndrome: A Biological Approach*; and J. Nijs and K. De Meirleir, Impairments of the 2-5A synthetase/RNase L pathway in CFS, *In Vivo* 19, no. 6 [Nov–Dec 2005] Review. A laboratory testing profile for CFS has just been developed at REDLABS USA. See www.redlabsusa.com.)

OXIDATIVE STRESS

A number of studies have now confirmed that CFS/FM patients generate more damaging free radicals than healthy controls. Free radicals are produced by all human beings as a by product of normal physiological processes. Free radicals have the potential to damage cells—this is called oxidative stress—but humans have an antioxidant system that normally keeps free radicals in check. As Dr. Logan will explain in the nutrition chapter, dietary antioxidants are an important part of this defense system.

In addition to generating more free radicals, research also indicates that patients also have a diminished antioxidant capacity—their antioxidant defense system is operating in a sub-par fashion. The result may be compromised cellular function, which can ultimately affect fatigue, cognition, mood, and pain. New research on the influence of mobile phones on oxidative stress may make you think twice about using a cell phone for extended periods.

CFS/FM patients often complain that they are sensitive to cell phones, computers, or so-called "electro-smog." Cellular phones and their base stations produce electromagnetic radiation. Some new research suggests that CFS/FM patients should reconsider cell phone use, or at least limit time spent on the phone. One of every two North Americans now uses a cellular phone. The voluntary exposure of the brain to microwaves from cell phones has been described by Dr. Leif Salford of Lund University, Sweden, as "the largest biologic experiment in the history of humankind." Studies in vitro have shown nerve cell damage to mammalian brain cells after exposure to frequencies emitted from cell phones. Recently, a study showed that cell phone use can cause negative impairments in cognitive function in otherwise healthy adults.

Even in the absence of acute symptoms from cell phones, new studies have shown that they can increase oxidative stress in both test tube and living animals. CFS/FM patients can ill afford an additional source of oxidative stress.

New generations of cell phones, such as those capable of transmitting internet data, may be even worse for CFS/FM patients. Radio signals for the next generation of mobile phones can cause headaches and nausea, according to a study conducted by three government ministries in Holland. The study compared the impact of radiation from base stations used for the current mobile telephone network with that of base stations for new third generation (3G) networks for fast data transfer, which will enable high-speed data services on a mobile device. The 3G base stations, compared to other bases, caused a significant rise in bodily complaints.

Cell phones can also open the blood-brain barrier in living systems and may allow potentially toxic material through this normally protective filtering system. A porous blood-brain barrier is thought to contribute to some of the neurological symptoms of CFS/FM. In addition, a porous blood-brain barrier may contribute to the sensitivities and intolerances to chemicals such as monosodium glutamate and aspartame.

If you must use a cell phone, use an air tube hands-free kit and keep the cell phone away from your body. If the phone and all the electronic components are further from your head, your exposure will be limited. Standard headset wires can double the amount of radiation exposure to the head and body, according to UK studies. The reason is that the wire connecting the cell phone to the ear/headset acts as an antenna. Air tube hands-free kits are available at the EMF SuperStore (www.lessemf.com) and may be worthwhile for certain CFS/FM patients. The EMF SuperStore is an excellent resource for those seeking to reduce total electro-smog exposure.

ELEVATED NITRIC OXIDE-PEROXYNITRITE THEORY

In 2000, our colleague Dr. Martin Pall of Washington State University published his theory explaining the vast array of symptoms of CFS/FM. Published in the journal *Medical Hypotheses*, his theory received considerable international attention. The elevated nitric oxide-peroxynitrite theory as the cause of CFS is quite complex, and a detailed review is beyond the scope of this book. However, exciting new research has backed up his ideas so an overview is worthwhile.

Basically, it goes like this: An infectious process, trauma, chemical exposure, or other triggering event leads to the release of inflammatory immune chemicals called cytokines. Inflammatory cytokines cause the release of nitric oxide (the bad kind, not the good kind called constitutive, which is enhanced by blood pressure medications and Viagra). Nitric oxide in turn reacts with a chemical called superoxide, leading to the formation of the explosive pro-oxidant called peroxynitrite. A continuous over-production of peroxynitrite is a significant burden for the body and a major contributor to oxidative stress and damage from free radicals. The problem in CFS/FM and MCS is that this process does not get shut down. In a vicious cycle, the peroxynitrite leads to more nitric oxide and so it continues, accounting for numerous symptoms throughout bodily systems. It is certainly exciting when a theory becomes validated, and the preliminary research thus far has supported the hypothesis.

A growing number of studies have confirmed that CFS patients are indeed under increased oxidative stress. A preliminary study published in the *Journal of Molecular Biochemistry* has confirmed that elevated peroxynitrite is a factor in ongoing CFS. Undoubtedly there will be further research into this area. The good news for patients is that the peroxynitrite theory also proposes effective treatments to cut off the cycle. Many of the nutritional interventions, botanicals, and dietary supplements discussed by Dr. Logan in the nutrition and dietary supplement chapters may prove to be helpful in lowering peroxynitrite and the overall oxidative stress burden. Fish oil (omega 3) concentrated in EPA, GLA from evening primrose oil, Efamol (omega 6), green tea, bilberry, ginger, licorice, and beneficial bacteria (probiotics) may all influence the peroxynitrite cycle. Although large-scale studies are required to fully explore the theory and potential interventions, the early data suggest that CFS/FM patients are burdened by elevated peroxynitrite and that dietary/supplemental antioxidants are of value.

NEW OXIDATIVE STRESS THEORY OF ME/CFS, MCS ETIOLOGY

The oxidative stress theory states that there is nitric-oxide-mediated stimulation of neurotransmitters with the release of glutamate and the inhibition of Cytochrome P-450 detoxification metabolism. As a result of peroxynitrite-mediated ATP depletion there is consequently hypersensitivity of NMDA receptors. The peroxynitrite-mediated increased permeability of the blood-brain barrier allows increased access of organic chemicals to the CNS, which could cause neural sensitization and multiple chemical sensitivity. (M. L. Paul, MDA sensitization and stimulation by peroxynitrite, nitric oxide, and organic solvents as the mechanism of chemical sensitivity in multiple chemical sensitivity, *Federation of American Societies for Experimental Biology Journal* 16, no. 11 [Sept 2002]: 1407–17.)

HEAVY METALS AND TOTAL BODY TOXIC BURDEN

The influence of heavy metals such as mercury and aluminum in CFS/FM has been debated for many years. There are some published scientific articles that warrant a discussion of mercury and aluminum within this text. A brief overview of mercury and aluminum is a good starting point.

Mercury

Methyl mercury is the organic and most toxic form of mercury. Large fish can accumulate significant amounts of mercury, and up to 95 percent is in the highly toxic methyl mercury form. Certain fish, including fresh tuna, swordfish, tilefish, and shark should be avoided by CFS/FM patients to avoid adding a methyl mercury burden. For a current assessment of the mercury in fish, see the Environmental Working Group Web site at www.ewg.org. Harvard Medical School research (*Archives of Pathology and Laboratory Medicine*, 2003) and independent testing from *Consumer Reports* (July 2003) shows that fish oil supplements are generally safe and free of mercury and other toxins. Consumers can examine the safety of fish oil supplements by examining the Web site—supplements that have passed the tests are listed and can be deemed safe for CFS/FM patients.

The influence of dental amalgams as a source of mercury toxicity has been investigated in a number of studies. There is no question that "silver" or mercury amalgam fillings release mercury vapor in the mouth as a result of chewing. In fact, a relationship between the number of fillings and the amount of mercury vapor within the mouth has been demonstrated. In addition, a number of studies have shown a connection between the number of fillings and mercury in saliva, blood, and urine. Chronic, low-level exposure to mercury has, however, been shown to cause vague symptoms similar to those of CFS/FM, including fatigue, headaches, cognitive difficulties, and muscle and/or joint pain. Even low levels of mercury, it turns out, can affect attention and fine motor skills in otherwise healthy adults. If this is the case in healthy individuals, it is likely compounded in CFS/FM patients. Some new physiological studies have uncovered why mercury wreaks havoc in the body, particularly the brain. Methyl mercury can easily pass through the blood-brain barrier, a protective network of blood vessels around the brain. Once inside the brain, methyl mercury is converted into inorganic mercury, where it hangs around for a long time—years in fact. Mercury in the body and in the central nervous system acts as a pro-oxidant or rusting agent at a biochemical level—i.e., it generates damaging free radicals. Mercury (and the number of dental amalgams) has been shown to markedly reduce the antioxidant activity in otherwise healthy adults. As previously discussed, a reduction in antioxidant activity in CFS/FM is a real problem. Given what we know about the antioxidant defense system in CFS/FM, patients can ill afford a further decrease in antioxidant activity.

Aluminum
The influence of aluminum, a potentially neurotoxic metal, on the development/course of Alzheimer's has been hotly debated.

Whether cause or effect, at this point it is clear that the absorption of aluminum from the gastrointestinal tract is increased in Alzheimer's disease. The sources of aluminum include water, food (particularly baking powder), antacids, and antiperspirants. Of these, food appears to be the most significant contributor to the aluminum burden. Those with Alzheimer's disease have been shown to have a threefold increase in the absorption of aluminum over healthy controls.

Although the absorption of aluminum from food, drink, and other sources has not been investigated in CFS/FM, a very important study published in the journal *Brain Research Bulletin* (2001) showed that CFS patients indeed have significantly increased blood aluminum. This research deserves follow-up and suggests that CFS patients have increased intestinal absorption of aluminum. It is known that aluminum can have detrimental effects on cognition and may indeed be a contributor to the cognitive deficits observed in CFS/FM.

Heavy Metal Detoxification in CFS/FM

Efforts to reduce the heavy metal burden in CFS/FM may be a worthwhile venture in those patients with this problem. It also may help to reduce some of the symptoms. Two studies published in the journal *Neuroendocrinology Letters* (1999, 2002) indicate that carefully supervised removal of amalgams, physician-guided detoxification, and antioxidant therapy can reduce the symptoms of CFS. In addition, a series of case reports published in the *Journal of Orthopaedic Medicine* (2001) showed that similar heavy metal detoxification protocols, when medically supervised, can reduce the symptoms of FM.

I need to emphasize that heavy metal detoxification should not be undertaken without supervision by a skilled practitioner. There are a number of prescription and non-prescription methods used to remove heavy metals from the body. This process is known as "chelation." A chelating agent is a chemical that is used as a preferential sponge to remove unwanted metals in the body. I was first exposed to the concept of chelation when I was a resident at the Hospital for Sick Children here in Toronto. An iron chelator called deferoxamine was used in the children who suffered from the hereditary anemia Thalassemia major. These children had severe anemia that was only treatable by ongoing blood transfusions of packed red blood cells. If they didn't have blood transfusions on a regular basis, they died at a very early age. In the past they lived longer as a result of the blood transfusions but died later of an accumulation of iron in their tissues as a result of the blood transfusions, often dying of heart failure or liver failure as a result of iron accumulation in their organs. A major breakthrough for these children began when they were chelated for excessive iron in their tissues. The medication deferoxamine was given slowly intravenously to remove the iron from their tissues after they received the blood transfusions. Their life expectancies increased considerably as a result of the chelation treatment.

Chelation is serious business and requires a gentle and knowledgeable approach. Simply removing amalgam fillings without supporting the body during the process with proper diet and nutrients/vitamins may become an expensive process that ultimately makes CFS/FM patients worse. During the removal of the mercury amalgams, some safety measures are needed both for your dentist and for you. You need a rubber dam, nasal oxygen, constant suction, and gauze under your tongue to collect mercury vapor that arises during the drilling process. Preferably your dentist will be familiar with environmental dentistry to protect himself, his staff, and you during the removal process. Everyone in the room except for the patient needs a full respirator face mask to prevent inhaling the mercury vapor. Ideally the mercury vapor should be vented outside the office so the rest of the staff do not inhale it and get contaminated by the mercury vapor. The dentist should use a high-speed drill so that the amalgam can be removed as quickly as possible. The longer the drilling occurs, the more mercury vapor is pouring into the air in the dentist's office.

In addition to the oral and possible intravenous nutrient protocols that may be advised, regular sauna therapy may be recommended. Sadly, medically induced sweating and sauna therapy is
a forgotten art. Research has documented that mercury and other
environmental toxins are present in, and excreted via, human
sweat. Using a sauna as a means to enhance the detoxification
process can be well worth the effort. Infrared sauna may be most
appropriate for CFS/FM detoxification and relaxation protocols
due to the gentle heating and comfortable environment. They
have been well tolerated by my patients with CFS/FM. Infrared
sauna therapy has been shown to improve circulation, and very
importantly for CFS/FM, to lower oxidative stress. Regular
saunas may not be as well tolerated by CFS/FM patients because
the heat is more intense and patients cannot stay in them for as
long. Relatively inexpensive infrared units are now available for
personal use at home, and due to the compact clip-together
design, they require little space. SaunaRay has an infrared sauna
that my patients have used. This company specifically manufac-
tures infrared saunas with materials friendly to chemically sensitive CFS/FM patients.

WHAT DO THE LAB RESULTS REALLY MEAN?

All of the various abnormalities documented in studies involving
CFS/FM patients may seem overwhelming. In addition, despite
all of the scientific results that appear to validate the existence of
the illnesses, there is still skepticism and a complete lack of a
diagnostic test. The specialized tests described above are just that,
specialized, and at this point in time they are available for
research only.

Patients should see hope in these exciting research results,
especially in the genetic studies. There are amazing people waking up every day all over this planet trying to uncover the mys-
teries of these illnesses. In research there is hope of treatment.
Every medical paper published showing that CFS/FM patients are
different from healthy controls—and different from those with

other medical conditions that involve fatigue and/or pain—provides validation that this is a physiologically based illness. If you are a CFS/FM patient, I'm sure you can relate to the fact that the average time from symptom presentation to diagnosis of CFS/FM is often five to seven years. Hopefully, the validation that comes through research will cut this timeframe dramatically so that those who follow will not have to endure this.

Lifestyle modifications, mind/body interventions, optimal nutrition, counseling, medications, nutrition, and some complementary therapies can tackle these documented abnormalities and associated symptoms to help with symptomatic relief of symptoms. At this time in CFS/FM research, the glass is half full with hope. Now let's move on to chapter 3 and get started with the helping!

CHAPTER THREE

PACING, ENERGY CONSERVATION, AND SLEEP HYGIENE

So if you have been diagnosed with CFS/FM and you want to improve your situation, pacing and energy conservation are now words to live by. According to research and my clinical experience, before you became ill you were probably a very active person, working full-time either inside or outside the home. Statistically, you are most likely a woman since more women are affected by these illnesses than men. But you may also be a child; children are also affected. It is likely that you were involved in many social or sporting activities and in general had a very busy life before you were sick.

However, you've probably also discovered that your old ways of coping by pushing yourself harder until you get things done now results in "crashing" or being bedridden for one to many days after you've pushed yourself. Your energy is likely 30 to 90 percent less than it was when you were healthy. You may be experiencing widespread body pain, extreme fatigue, and a host of other symptoms in many body systems. This is the world of CFS/FM. The key now is to focus on how you can improve and begin your road to recovery.

For most of us, our means of coping though life has been to push . . . doing a bit more, being a bit more, ultimately pushing ourselves to bits. Trying to do it "all," be it "all," and please everyone "all" the time. Wow, I get tired just thinking about "all" of this. This coping mechanism is not only ineffective, it is actually destructive when you have CFS/FM. It's also destructive when you are healthy. *No one* can do it "all"! There is no such thing as a superwoman or superman. So give this idea up for good, for your good health.

I am now going to teach you about *energy conservation*, both physical and emotional. Energy conservation is not a new principle to medicine; it is based on the occupational therapy model that has been applied to arthritis, multiple sclerosis, and many chronic illnesses. I first learned about it years ago when I was at a conference on CFS in Dublin, Ireland. It was like a light bulb going off for me. My patients kept talking about pushing and crashing and I was intrigued enough to try something new. I took the concepts home to Toronto. I said to my patients, "You already know how to push and that it results in crashing. How would you like to try something new called energy conservation?" After trying these therapies, I found them to be some of the most successful tools I have been able to teach my patients. I have patients keep a daily diary or activity log and use this plus the functional capacity scale to determine their level of functioning.

ACTIVITY LOG

My role as a medical doctor is multifaceted. In this situation, my role is to teach people how to pace themselves. I see myself as the coach and the patient as the player on my team—if they wish to join. I really focus on the principles of pacing because it allows patients to take control of their health in order to try to help them get better. When I originally see patients, they are in what is called the crashing pattern (see the sample normal and crashing activity logs on the following pages).

A normal person has a good night's sleep and feels refreshed, (very good sleep quality—level 5). She can do activities all day

---

Your Activity Log:
- Keep it in a handy place.
- Complete it every day.
- Take your completed logs to your doctor/health care provider at follow-up visits.
- Your logs assist your doctor in adjusting your treatment plan as needed.
- Completed logs may reassure your insurance company of your active ongoing participation in your treatment.

Completing Your Activity Log:
- You may change the times on the lefthand side of the log to suit your usual schedule (e.g., if you usually get up at 10:00 a.m. and go to bed at 2:00 a.m., write 10:00 a.m. in as the first time and adjust the other times accordingly).
- Note your activities with one or two word(s) in the appropriate time slots (e.g., dressed, made bed, took nap).
- Rest is defined as lying down, with eyes shut, meditating or sleeping.

Figure 1. Activity log for a "normal" patient.

Name **Normal** _____ Date _____

Day	Monday	Tuesday	Wednesday	Thursday	Friday	Saturday	Sunday
Number of hours slept between 11:00 p.m. and 6:00 a.m.	5	5	5	5	5	5	5
Sleep Quality (1: very poor; 2: poor; 3: fair; 4: good; 5: very good)							
Functional Capacity Scale at Beginning of Day: 0–10							
Activities (please specify)							
6:00 a.m.							
7:00 a.m.	9	9	9	9	10	9	9
8:00 a.m.							
9:00 a.m.							
10:00 a.m.							
11:00 a.m.							
12:00 p.m.							
1:00 p.m.							
2:00 p.m.							
3:00 p.m.							
4:00 p.m.							
5:00 p.m.							
6:00 p.m.							
7:00 p.m.							
8:00 p.m.							
9:00 p.m.							
10:00 p.m.							
11:00 p.m.							
Number of minutes walked/day		60		60		60	60
Number of usable hours/day							
Functional Capacity Scale at End of Day: 0–10	9	9	9	9	9	9	9

Figure 2. Activity log for a patient in a crashing pattern.

Name **Crashing pattern** _____ Date _____

Day	Monday	Tuesday	Wednesday	Thursday	Friday	Saturday	Sunday
Number of hours slept between 11:00 p.m. and 6:00 a.m.	4	4	4	2	2	2	3
Sleep Quality (1: very poor; 2: poor; 3: fair; 4: good; 5: very good)							
Functional Capacity Scale at Beginning of Day: 0–10							
Activities (please specify)							
6:00 a.m.							
7:00 a.m.							
8:00 a.m.							
9:00 a.m.							
10:00 a.m.	4	4	5	3	3	3	4
11:00 a.m.							
12:00 p.m.							
1:00 p.m.							
2:00 p.m.							
3:00 p.m.							
4:00 p.m.							
5:00 p.m.							
6:00 p.m.							
7:00 p.m.							
8:00 p.m.							
9:00 p.m.							
10:00 p.m.							
11:00 p.m.							
Number of minutes walked/day	10	10	20	0	0	0	0
Number of usable hours/day							
Functional Capacity Scale at End of Day: 0–10	3	3	2	2	2	2	2

long and has normal energy of 9 in the morning and in the evening 9 as well. Normal energy (the white areas of the log) is 9 or 10 out of 10 according to the Functional Capacity Scale (see page 62). Normal people can occasionally stay up all night tending a sick child and still go to work the next day without any difficulties. They can exercise for sixty minutes three times a week with ease.

Figure 2 is typical of a patient in the crashing pattern with CFS/FM. On a good day their energy (the light grey areas) is 4 out of 10. They need rest periods throughout the day. Their energy drops by 1 point to 3 by the end of the day when their energy is lowest. They have an occasional good day—in this case, Wednesday—with a better energy level of 5 and they do not rest because they feel so good. As a result they crash over the next three days: their energy drops to their low level of 3 and they spend most of the next three days resting. The patient cannot walk on many days because they are too exhausted. Rest and sleep are indicated in dark grey.

Crashing means that if you do too much one day, the next day (or the next several days to a week or more) you end up crashing and spending time in bed with greatly reduced energy. The pattern I see with most patients is they do too much and then crash. They repeat this pattern again and again. Over a period of time, if they continue with this pattern, their energy level gets worse and worse.

So, in my office, one of the roles I assume is that of a coach to help patients make lifestyle changes. So if I am the coach, then the patient is the player. What this means is that I can teach you the principles of the game, but you are the one that has to do the work and make the lifestyle changes to try to improve your health. Joining a well-run education and support group can be valuable. At the office we have an educational support group that is based on the Harvard Mind-Body course. I offer this course together with the naturopathic doctor who works with me at my office, Dr. Tracey Beaulne. The group setting works well to rein-

Figure 3. Activity log for a patient in a recovery pattern.

Name **Recovery pattern** _____ Date _____

Day	Monday	Tuesday	Wednesday	Thursday	Friday	Saturday	Sunday
Number of hours slept between 11:00 p.m. and 6:00 a.m.	4	4	4	4	4	4	4
Sleep Quality (1: very poor; 2: poor; 3: fair; 4: good; 5: very good)							
Functional Capacity Scale at Beginning of Day: 0–10							
Activities (please specify)							
6:00 a.m.							
7:00 a.m.							
8:00 a.m.	6	6	6	6	6	6	6
9:00 a.m.							
10:00 a.m.							
11:00 a.m.							
12:00 p.m.							
1:00 p.m.							
2:00 p.m.							
3:00 p.m.							
4:00 p.m.							
5:00 p.m.							
6:00 p.m.							
7:00 p.m.							
8:00 p.m.							
9:00 p.m.							
10:00 p.m.							
11:00 p.m.							
Number of minutes walked/day	20	20	20	20	20	20	20
Number of usable hours/day							
Functional Capacity Scale at End of Day: 0–10	5	5	5	5	5	5	5

force the principles we teach. This book covers many of the educational topics we cover in the group setting. Patients feel supported in the group because they come together with others who have similar problems and they are no longer alone. They often form valuable friendships that last for many years. They are given and also share valuable information about available resources in their communities such as places for aquatherapy, volunteer transportation organizations, etc.

I try to teach my patients the recovery pattern (see figure 3). With CFS/FM, "recovery" involves advance planning or planning ahead of time. What this means is that you rest *before* and *after* activities so that you avoid crashing at any cost. This has been referred to as "aggressive rest therapy." Rest in this case means lying down with your eyes shut, either sleeping or meditating. Rest does not mean watching TV or reading. Both watching TV and reading burn about 150 calories an hour. The brain is engaged and energy is being used during both of these activities. Only while resting do the brain and the body have a chance to heal.

The most important feature of the recover pattern of activity is the ongoing rest periods that are planned during the hours of better energy. By doing this, patients do not crash and have more consistent energy levels so that they can begin to plan their activities. The most important activity to plan is some sort of exercise. In this chart the patient can walk for twenty minutes on most days and start to rebuild their muscles.

This principle of resting applies to you regardless of whether you are mildly, moderately, or severely disabled. By allowing some time for healing throughout the day, your crashes become fewer and farther apart and eventually you do not crash at all if you continue to listen to your body and stop before you are exhausted. The energy that you would have put toward a crash is now available for healing, and your health gradually improves. What usually results is a slow incremental increase of energy and you begin to have better energy during part of the day. This improves and eventually becomes the occasional good day. These good days are like pearls. Eventually you get more good days and those pearls form an entire necklace of good health.

These gains happen slowly and in small increments on the road to recovery. In my practice, I have patients who have been severely disabled for many years. Even these patients can experience improvement and relief of many symptoms. One patient who had been ill for more than ten years and unable to work learned how to pace. A few years later she was able to work part-time as a teacher.

When patients apply the principles of pacing, they get a better, more consistent energy level, and they have a better quality of life. When their energy is better they can begin to plan activities ahead of time and to keep their plans. Energy conservation is a way to accomplish life's ongoing tasks without making yourself sicker. It is a strategy to balance your life between doing the things you want to do and resting appropriately.

Central to the pacing principle is the maintenance of an activity log. This is a diary just like your planning diary that you used while you worked full time. It is a compact way of keeping track of your activities. Every hour on the hour you write down what you are doing. You record your sleep hours and quality of your sleep. You also record your energy levels from 0 to 10 at the best time of the day (most often in the morning) and the worst time of the day (most often the evening) according to the functional capacity scale.

FUNCTIONAL CAPACITY SCALE

I came up with the idea for this Functional Capacity Scale (see page 62) because a number of patients were reporting significant improvements and based on their improvements I thought that they were ready to try and return to work. They would proceed back to work, only to have a total relapse of their symptoms in two or three months. I would see them back in consultation, and we would both be puzzled by what happened and why they suddenly couldn't work when we had thought they would be able to. What I discovered was that often people felt much better but their energy was not sustainable or reliable on an ongoing daily basis. I needed a tool to help me, and at the time there wasn't one available.

The Functional Capacity Scale crystallized for me even more after my own personal health experiences. I became severely ill with pneumococcal meningitis about eight years ago. I ended up in the hospital's Intensive Care Unit unconscious and off work for a long time. As a result of my own recovery, I was able to gain firsthand appreciation of severe fatigue and cognitive difficulties. Fortunately, I have fully recovered, but my illness allowed me a much better understanding of severe disability, even though I myself was only disabled for a relatively short period of time.

The Functional Capacity Scale ranges from zero to ten. The scale is divided into two elements—physical and cognitive. Zero represents no energy at all, totally bedridden and unable to do even self-care or bathe yourself. In this situation a bed bath would be required. This energy level would represent a patient who was in the ICU or had just undergone major surgery.

At the other end of the scale is 9 out of 10, which would be considered normal for most people. *Normal* means, in terms of activity, the person can work full time (forty to fifty hours a week) and have a full social life, including exercising three to five times a week, and socializing on the weekends. This means that the person can function fully for sixteen hours a day continuously, without becoming fatigued and requiring a nap or a period where they must lie down to rest. Most people can skip the occasional full night of sleep and manage to get through the next day's activities without difficultly.

An energy level of 10 out of 10 would represent that small percentage of individuals like William the Conqueror and the former Prime Minister of Great Britain, Lady Margaret Thatcher, who require very little sleep at night, often only four or five hours. These people have extremely high energy and very little sleep requirements, and as a result they may become great leaders. Most people function about 9 out of 10 most of the time. Fatigue to a normal person means that they get the feeling of being tired, so they sit down for fifteen or twenty minutes or lie down and have a twenty-minute power nap and feel raring to go as soon as they get up.

This scale came about as a result of the multiple uses of the word *fatigue* in our society. It is a very poorly defined term and, as mentioned, one person's fatigue is not necessarily another's fatigue when it comes to impairment of health and diminished physical activity. I had real difficulties with patients trying to figure out just exactly how fatigued they were because sometimes if you feel "fatigued" you are able to perform physical activities, and other times if you feel "fatigued" you are totally bedridden.

You can find blank activity logs and the functional capacity scale online at the Ontario College of Family Physicians Web site at: www.ocfp.on.ca/english/ocfp/communications/publications/default.asp?s=1#EnvironmentHealth. Please feel free to copy them for your own use and to take copies to your doctor for his or her use with other patients.

When I review patients' activity logs, I can see what they are doing each hour of each day, the times they are doing it, and the effect that it has on them. The energy levels present at the best (usually morning) and worst (usually evening) times of the day are scored by using numbers from the Functional Capacity Scale. In some patients, energy is best near the end of the day and worst at the beginning of the day. The pattern of energy is always the same for a particular patient; it does not flip back and forth.

People with CFS/FM are different from healthy individuals when it comes to planning physical activity. They must rest before and after an activity, not so that they feel raring to go, but so that they can just manage not to get worse. If they do push themselves and don't rest throughout the day, inevitably they use up more energy than they have and they crash. The next one to three days may lead to an incapacitated state, totally bedridden,

FUNCTIONAL CAPACITY SCALE

The Functional Capacity Scale incorporates energy rating, symptom severity, and activity level. The description after each scale number should help you to rate your functional capacity at the beginning and end of each day.

0   No energy, severe symptoms including very poor concentration; bed-ridden all day; cannot do self-care (need bed bath to be given).

1   Severe symptoms at rest, including very poor concentration; in bed most of the day; need assistance with self-care activities.

2   Severe symptoms at rest, including poor concentration; frequent rests or naps; need some assistance with limited self-care activities.

3   Moderate symptoms at rest, including poor concentration; need frequent rests or naps; can do independent self-care but have severe post-exertion fatigue.

4   Moderate symptoms at rest, including some difficulty concentrating; need frequent rests throughout the day; can do independent self-care and limited activities of daily living (e.g,. light housework, laundry); can walk for a few minutes per day.

5   Mild symptoms at rest with fairly good concentration for short periods (fifteen minutes); need a.m. and p.m. rest; can do independent self-care and moderate activities of daily living, but have slight post-exertion fatigue; can walk ten to twenty minutes per day.

6   Mild or no symptoms at rest with fairly good concentration for up to 45 minutes, cannot multitask; need afternoon rest; can do most activities of daily living except vacuuming; can walk twenty to thirty minutes per day; can do volunteer work—maximum total time four hours per week, with flexible hours.

7   Mild or no symptoms at rest with good concentration for up to half a day; can do more intense activities of daily living (e.g., grocery shopping, vacuuming) but may get post-exertion fatigue if "overdo": can walk thirty minutes per day; can work limited hours, less than twenty-five hours per week; no or minimal social life.

8   Mild intermittent symptoms with good concentration; can do full self-care, work forty hours per week, enjoy a social life, do moderate vigorous exercise three times per week.

9   No symptoms with very good concentration, full work and social life; can do vigorous exercise three to five times a week.

10 No symptoms, excellent concentration, over achiever (sometimes may require less sleep than average person).

NUMBER OF USABLE HOURS PER DAY = Number of hours NOT asleep or resting/meditating with eyes closed.

Dr. Lynn Marshall, Co-Author, Director, Environmental Health Clinic, Sunnybrook & Women's College Health Services Centre

© Dr. Alison Bested

PLEASE FEEL FREE TO COPY THE FUNCTIONAL CAPACITY SCALE AND USE IT.

rising only for meals. It becomes an effort to recover energy to the previous level.

ENERGY AS MONEY

I use mental imagery with my patients to help them learn the limits of their energy, especially when they first come to me. Most patients can relate to the concept of energy as money. This idea was from the work of Dr. Darrel Ho-Yen and was presented in the book *Better Recovery from Viral Illnesses* (Dodona Books, 1999). An expert in chronic fatigue syndrome, Dr. Ho-Yen explains that you should think of today's energy as cash. This energy money is all the energy you have to live on for one day. When you have CFS/FM, you have a huge loan and are in debt to the energy bank. If you use more than today's cash amount, you crash. Yesterday's energy check has been cashed and is worthless and

HERMAN®

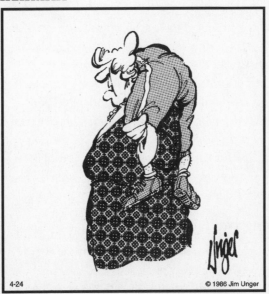

4-24   © 1986 Jim Unger

**"I'm not going through this every
time you go jogging."**

tomorrow's check is a post-dated check that may not come. The best thing that you can do is to try and live each day in the moment. Live within the limits of the energy that you do have.

On a particularly good day, it's best not to use up all of your energy by trying to make up for all previously unfinished business or projects. Instead, try to "pay down" some of your outstanding energy loan. What this means is that even on a good day you should stay in the same routine and plan it out as if it were any other day. When you don't overdo it on a good day, the increased energy and lowered pain will ultimately help to pay back your physical and mental energy loan. Patients who manage their energy loan will improve at a faster rate than those who don't. In CFS/FM there is no such thing as "overdraft protection." Although it's tempting, don't try to squeeze everything in on that one good day when you have good energy and/or lower pain. If you do try to "do it all" on a good day, I guarantee you will crash.

THE RECHARGEABLE BATTERY

Another mental image to keep in mind is to see your body as a battery. You have only so much energy, and once your battery is dead you crash. Let's say that you are operating on energy levels of 6 out of 10, or that your battery has 60 percent of its energy. This means that you can use a maximum of 60 percent energy on a given day, but to go beyond puts you in a place where the recovery process is on hold and may cause a set-back or worsening of symptoms. In this case you have drained your battery dry. If you take your rest periods throughout the day, you will keep your battery charged up and avoid crashing.

GLASS BOX IMAGE

The other way I ask patients to visualize their energy is to visualize themselves completely enclosed inside a glass box. If they listen to their bodies, they will learn the limits of their box and stay within it. As a result, their box will slowly expand as their health improves. On a good day when this box expands, they are able to do a few more activities. They still have cycles of good and bad days but they stay within the limits of their energy box. However, if they have a good day and use up all of their energy and push themselves to do more (as they used to do when they were well), they will smash through their glass box and bleed all over the floor (metaphorically speaking). Their glass box will shrink to a much smaller size than before. They will have crashed. They will have no energy to heal their illness; all their energy will be tied up in trying to recover from the most recent crash.

Unfortunately I have seen patients continue to push and crash until they have become bedridden to the point where they require full-time care in a residential facility—otherwise known as a nursing home. This is not a great place to be if you are middle aged. Why in a nursing home? Because there is no other place available to deal with this degree of care on a long-term chronic basis.

So at their follow-up visits, patients bring their activity logs with them for me to review. On their activity logs, they have filled the spaces with words recording their actual activities, such as resting, folding laundry, meals, watching TV, walking, etc. I can see the crashing pattern on their log. I point the pattern out if they have not recognized it themselves, but most do see the crashes after doing too much. For example, if they had a very low energy, say 3 out of 10, and they tried to do one outside activity such as shopping or going to the doctor's office two days in a row without having a quieter day at home in between, they would likely crash. The next two to three days would probably be spent in bed, only getting up for meals.

When I review patients' activity logs at each visit, I point out to them the effects of the way they are scheduling their activities on their body. If, for example, their energy level was 5 and they crashed with two outside activities on one day, I would suggest they plan only one outside activity each day and see if their energy supports them without crashing.

The activity logs become an important tool to help patients

see the effects of their activities on their fatigue and other symptoms. At first patients can use them to learn how to avoid crashing. In order to do this they need to learn to listen to their body and what messages are being given that can guide them. Many patients, when they come to me, are brain driven and body dead. Their brains were writing checks that their bodies could not cash. Individual patients must learn their body's signal to know when to stop. This is one of the tools or keys for learning how to avoid a crash. For some patients, it might be that they feel a sore throat coming on. Others may get a raspy voice. Many get "brain fog," while others feel as if all of their energy has gone down the sewer. Individual patients almost always experience the same symptom time and again. Learning your body's signal or symptom is cluing in your thinking brain to what your unconscious brain (that controls body processes) is doing. This is what mind-body medicine is all about: being "body aware" in the moment. It is nothing new; some of us have simply blocked it out except for rare emergencies.

MOBILITY AND EXERCISE

CFS/FM patients have lost muscle mass as a result of their severe fatigue and immobility. Consequently they are at risk for developing osteoporosis or osteopenia. Patients need to keep as active as possible. They need to use their muscles as often as possible to keep the muscles that they do have and to build new muscles to rebuild their strength and improve their energy. The key is to rebuild the muscle mass without crashing. The principles are the same no matter your energy level.

So if you are bedridden and are using a commode (bedside toilet), start by doing some range of motion exercises while you are in bed. This means that you move your arms and legs in all the directions they can go while you are in bed. By putting your limbs through their full range of motion, you slowly gain muscle strength and also prevent muscle shortening or contracture. Take your arms, for example; they go above your head, down to your sides, across your chest, out to your sides, and behind you. Start with one range of motion arm exercise on the first day. The next day do the leg range of motion exercise. Make sure that you can manage the exercise before you try to do too much. Always start with what you know you can do; it's always better to start exercising *below* what you can do. In other words: *start low and go slow*. If you have access to a physiotherapist to design a program of exercises for you, this is even better. However, remember that it's your body and you know its limits better than anyone, so if you think the exercises are too much for you, only do one or two repetitions to begin with. It's better to start with too little and gradually build up the number of repetitions than to do too many repetitions and crash as a result.

If you are mostly bedridden and can walk to the bathroom, can you walk to the bathroom a second time and not crash? Can you do this more than once a day? Every little bit helps.

If you are housebound most of the time, it is often helpful to wear a pedometer to count the number of steps you take each day. If you know how many steps you take on an average day and you would like to do more, I recommend the 10 percent rule, which is simply adding 10 percent more steps to your daily total. So if you now walk, say, 1,000 steps, and you are improving, add an additional 100 steps to your daily in-house walking for a period of time of one week. You should be able to do this and avoid crashing that day. Learn to walk inside your house by doing *perimeter walking*.

The idea of perimeter walking came to me as I watched the animals at our nearby Metro Toronto Zoo. The animals have spacious outside areas that they live in as well as inside living quarters. Their spaces are surrounded by fences, and the animals are often seen getting their exercise by walking around the perimeter of the enclosure just inside the fence.

You can do your own perimeter walking by walking just inside the walls of your house or apartment. Just go from room to room on the same floor walking close to the walls. I do not suggest that you climb the stairs at this point, it takes too much energy. If you live in an apartment building and you are safe, you can walk up and down your hallway. Use a kitchen timer or a watch with a second hand so that you know exactly how many minutes you have walked. This is important to keep track of so that if you walk outside your home you don't overdo it and end up crashing.

If your balance is poor, as is the case with many patients, use a walker for stability. It is best if you purchase a walker that has wheels, breaks, a seat, and a basket. It should be measured for your height and weight. This way you can sit down for little breaks during your walk time. If you are more steady on your feet but need help some of the time, consider a cane that has been specifically fitted to your hand that is ergonomically correct so that you do not increase your hand and wrist pain every time you walk. To prevent accidental falls, always use hand rails when going up and down stairs. Also, always wear your best support shoes from the time you get up in the morning until you go to bed at night. Your feet and legs need the support. It helps to prevent pain in the soles of your feet, or plantar fasciitis. It also keeps you more steady on your feet and prevents falls.

If you want to get out of the house for a change of scenery but are not up to walking, consider going to a nearby mall and renting a wheelchair while one of your friends or family pushes you. This way you can enjoy the outing without crashing in bed the next couple of days. You may not want anyone to see you in a wheelchair, but my advice to you is park your pride at home. You can always pick it up later, after you have enjoyed being out without crashing. Try it just once and see if you don't enjoy yourself and forget about being embarrassed after the first few minutes. But remember; don't stay out too long the first time. You will spend a lot of energy just looking around at things in the mall. Energy is more than simply physical, as you have no doubt already discovered.

If you are able to walk ten minutes outside the house and

wish to increase, by using the 10 percent rule you would add one minute to your walking routine. It isn't much, but it is an incremental improvement that you can manage without crashing.

The key is to be consistent in your exercise so that you gradually rebuild your muscles, increasing slowly at your own rate. If you do not recover the same day and you have post-exertional fatigue the next day, you have done too much for the energy available to you. When you walk, I suggest that you walk on level ground without hills or stairs. If you are walking uphill you need more energy than walking on level ground (higher aerobic activity). This is often too intense for patients, but they often do not even notice when they are walking on an incline. If you are starting to feel a little strained, look back behind you and see if you are walking uphill and didn't notice it before.

If you are able to walk for fifteen to twenty minutes, it is time to start doing some strength training exercises on a regular basis. I recommend the book *Strong Women Stay Young* by Miriam Nelson. It was written specifically for women who suffer from osteoporosis. It is a marvelous book with easy-to-understand pictures and descriptions on how to do the exercises correctly. The book divides the exercises into four upper body and four lower body exercises. The exercises must be done slowly to a count of four with time in the middle of the repetition to breathe. Proper technique is extremely important when doing strength training exercises. Ideally you should be taught individually by a physiotherapist or personal trainer, but this is not available to most people as it can be very expensive. The book is a great alternative with some modifications for the CFS/FM population.

Start your strength training program by doing only three repetitions without using any weights. I want to stress this—*no weights*. When patients start out right at the beginning using weights, they often strain their tendons and are in pain and unable to use their strained muscles for a couple of months afterward. If patients didn't have muscle pain before, they do now. So please, be very careful when you start strength training and begin

> ## The Ground Rules for Physical Activity
> - Small changes over time, a gradual process
> - 10 percent rule
> - Learn new ways to do things
> - Even something small is better than nothing
> - Be super-cautious about the "good days"
> - Rest during your good energy and poor energy times to recharge your battery
> - Find what type of physical activity works for you
> - Use your energy wisely, prevent crashing, and begin recovery

with only three repetitions and no weights. It is always easy to increase the number of repetitions later when you know you can do the exercises without crashing. Normal people can start doing eight repetitions and a few pounds of weight. You are not normal if you have CFS/FM.

I suggest breaking the exercises into upper body and lower body and keeping track of the exercises in a journal. Do the upper body exercises on Monday, and Thursday. Do the lower body exercises on Tuesday and Friday. You cannot do weight-bearing

HERMAN®

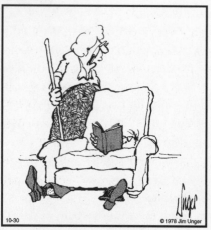

10-30   © 1978 Jim Unger

"You in one of your moods again?"

exercises every day. Your body needs time off in between so that new muscle can grow as a result of the weight-bearing exercise. From experience I find that twice a week is the most that patients can manage on a regular basis.

If you think you can do more repetitions, then I suggest you add one repetition for at least a couple of weeks before you add more. Your body needs time to adjust, and it is always better to go slowly so that you avoid crashing.

If you become ill or cannot exercise for a while, you will lose some of your muscle mass and strength within a few days. So reduce the time you walk or reduce the amount of weights and repetitions and begin again. Expect that you will begin again and again and again on your road to recovery. Do not get discouraged by this, but look back at your progress over time. This is where it really helps to keep your activity and exercise logs. Most often you will see that you have kept some of the gains you have made previously and now that you have learned how not to crash, you will keep more. Try to always compare yourself to where you were when you were the sickest during your illness. This will help to show you the tremendous gains you have made since that time.

After you have completed your exercises it is very important that you stretch your warm muscles. Do not stretch cold muscles because you can damage them. Often with the muscle pain of CFS/FM stretching is painful. Even so, in the long run it helps your muscles to regain their normal function if you stretch them on an ongoing basis. Some of my patients stretch their muscles throughout the day. Just remember to warm them up first. If you can't exercise, then get into a hot bath with Epsom salts or use a hot water bottle or hot pack first. Patients have reported that the following muscle treatment therapies are helpful: physiotherapy, chiropractic, acupuncture, aquatherapy, steam baths, saunas, massage therapy, Tai Chi, Qigong, Reiki, or therapeutic touch.

In essence you must learn new ways of doing things, because

the old ways no longer work. The key to getting on the road to recovery is finding a balance between small increases in activity and the prevention of setbacks or crashing.

DEALING WITH THE EMOTIONAL UPSETS THAT RESULT FROM CHRONIC ILLNESS

It is initially extremely difficult to follow the pacing and energy conservation principles because we live in a society that teaches us to push ourselves. It is especially hard not to push yourself on a good day or during the good time of the day when you have a little bit more energy. It's so tempting to use up all of your energy because you want to get all the things done that you normally couldn't do on a very low energy day.

The activity log not only addresses the physical changes that need to be made, it also forces CFS/FM patients to realize the reduced activity level that they actually have. Many patients are shocked and distressed because they have not reflected on daily activity levels and patterns. They often have not had the energy to do so. The activity log is a means to allow patients to recognize the emotional ramifications of having a chronic illness. For the first time, many patients can begin to address their denial of having a chronic illness and the influence of physical and mental exertion in their fatigue. Only through identifying their emotions can emotional issues be properly addressed and treated.

All patients with chronic illness, including CFS/FM patients, go through an emotional process as a result of having a life-altering medical condition. These are the same emotional reactions or stages that terminal cancer patients go through. They are outlined in *On Death and Dying*, by Dr. Kubler-Ross (Touchstone Press, 1997).

As part of helping patients cope with their chronic illness, I help them deal with their emotions. They go through various stages that last from a few months to many years in some patients. They flip back and forth through the stages throughout their illness. It is not a steady progression by any means. The emotional stages are denial, anger, depression, bargaining, and finally acceptance. In my experience, the activity logs, and the changes they initiate, are a means to address the denial phase and help the patient progress to a healthier emotional state.

Often when their energy is very low, patients are in what I call "survival mode." There is not enough energy to process emotions. When their energy improves to a 5 or 6 out of 10 they often begin to develop a reactive depression in response to being chronically ill. I call this a positive negative. It means that their energy has improved and now they have enough energy to begin to realize just how sick they really are. At this point they benefit from cognitive behavioral therapy to help them realistically grieve the losses of their jobs, finances, and often relationships that have resulted from their chronic illness. Dr. Jack Birnbaum taught me cognitive behavioral therapy in a group setting. This helps patients deal with the emotional stress of being chronically ill. I find the group setting is more effective because patients learn that they all have similar problems and get the support from one another. Often acknowledging their pain is the most helpful therapy and allowing them to express their grief in a healthy way is extremely beneficial. I often suggest patients watch the movie *Tuesdays with Morrie* for this purpose. It is an inspiring true story about a professor who comes to terms with the loss of his body's function as a result of Lou Gehrig's disease. It was written by Mitch Albom, who was a former student of Morrie's. The book was a result of weekly visits that Mitch made to Morrie's house every Tuesday. One of the things that Morrie did was to come to terms with his losses of body function over time. He did this by allowing himself a twenty-minute weeping spell every morning to grieve the losses he endured. When the twenty minutes were over he stopped himself from continuing to cry and carried on with the rest of his day the best he could. I encourage patients to do this when they get to the stage when they need to grieve the losses that have resulted from being chronically ill. Grief is a painful but necessary part of recovery. If grief is not expressed it may develop into depression over the long run. Another helpful book that looks at the spiritual side of chronic illness and the search for meaning is *Close to the Bone* by Jean Shinoda Bolen. Patients may need individual or group counseling at this point in their illness. If they do develop a reactive depression they may also benefit from carefully administered therapies including therapeutic levels of omega 3 fish oils and/or antidepressants.

Initially, keeping an activity log may provoke in patients a lot of negative reactions as they move through the emotions of denial, anger, and depression. Patients often do not like keeping them and really resist this task. I try to encourage my pateients to keep doing the activity logs regardless of their negative feelings toward them. The long-term goal is to use the activity log as a template for scheduling activities and rests. In essence, the activity log is ideally to be used as a planner so that patients learn how to best maximize their activities and minimize their pain and fatigue symptoms. It helps patients to develop a healthy routine. Some patients catch on to the principles extremely quickly, while others need years of encouragement to make these often-difficult lifestyle changes.

On the activity log, in addition to writing down what you are doing on an hourly basis, it is also important to document your functional capacity scale number at the best and worst time of the day. I also ask patients to write down how many total minutes they are able to walk during the day—this may include just one small walk of five or ten minutes or even the number of steps on their daily pedometer. Activities such as walking to the corner store for a loaf of bread or walking the dog should be included in this total number of minutes walked as well. In addition, I ask people to record on the activity log the number of hours they sleep and the quality of their sleep. I use a scale from zero to five for the quality of their sleep with zero being terrible and five being a restorative sleep. This lets me know if poor sleep is an issue for each patient. It usually is. I find that if patients do not sleep and do not get help with their sleep, their recovery is much slower.

Patients who keep activity logs and gradually make the lifestyle changes that include resting before an activity often have gradual improvements in their energy levels. This is not seen from week to week, but rather over a longer period of time up to six months to a year depending on the severity of their fatigue. CFS/FM patients also find that as they progress, keeping the activity log allows them to look back to see how they are doing now compared to how they were when they initially came to see me. I often find that because patients have cognitive problems that come with their illness, they often forget just how severe their symptoms were at the beginning. Appreciation of even the smallest gains is crucial to their recovery efforts. If you follow the program outlined in this book, clinical experience and medical research indicate that improvement is possible. Keeping the logs allows for recognition of even small gains made over time. Personal documentation of your life on the activity logs will become a real source of encouragement for you to see your own progress. This helps you with coping on your "bad" days.

PROGNOSIS

It has been recognized that the earlier the CFS/FM diagnosis is made and the milder the initial illness, the better the possibility is for full recovery. This is because undiagnosed patients continue to push themselves over and over again so that by the time they are finally diagnosed by someone like me, many years later, their energy levels are often down to two or three. If diagnosed early, often patients' energy levels have only slipped to 6 out of 10. It is much easier for the body to heal from the energy level of a 6 than from a 2 or 3.

My goal as a treating doctor is to help the patient to improve incrementally, one symptom at a time. Improving one symptom even slightly helps to decrease the entire body load and promotes healing one step at a time. Many doctors get frustrated when treating this illness because they want to heal the patient totally. I have learned to enjoy the small gains in symptoms such as improved sleep, more manageable pain, and improvements in energy over time. By looking for these incremental improvements, I show patients the improvement of their symptoms and the gains they have made in their illness and show them that they are improving and healing with time and effort on their part. This helps to keep their hope alive and they are usually uplifted after they have had an office visit with me.

The problem with ongoing CFS/FM research studies is that the degree of fatigue or disability is not measured when the person is entered into a study using either a functional capacity scale or a disability scoring scale. There is such a wide variation within the physical and mental limitations of patients being studied. As a result, the long-term effects of the study in terms of the prognosis are often not comparable because CFS/FM patients in one study may have an energy level of 6 or 7 and in another study may have an energy level of 2 or 3. It's like comparing apples and oranges. This problem can be addressed by using a uniform functional measuring scale to measure patients' abilities both physically and cognitively, allowing for a more accurate assessment of prognosis and recovery. This uniform functional measuring scale is currently being developed.

What I aim for in my practice is to help patients improve their ability to cope with their illness, care for themselves, and care for their family. If they are at an energy level of 3 or below, the goal is to get them functioning at a higher level. How high I cannot predict. The person may not recover fully. However, over time I find that people do learn new skills and their energy levels do gradually increase. Often they can have a better family and social life. Some can do volunteer work. For the fortunate few who get diagnosed early—within the first year—and have a milder form of the illness, I often find there can be recovery as long as the patient maintains mind-body awareness and does not crash because she has learned to stop pushing herself. One of the goals of this book, then, is to help patients get diagnosed earlier so they have a better chance of recovery. The more people out there that know about this illness, the better chances are that a diagnosis will be made earlier. Currently in my practice I tend to see more severely disabled patients because I am a doctor of last resort. Also CFS/ME is still poorly understood and little is known about it by doctors practicing medicine currently. This has improved a great deal compared to when I first began in this area of medicine, but we still have a long way to go. My long-term goal is to put myself out of business so that eventually CFS/FM will be diagnosed much earlier and patients will be treated sooner (by new and not-yet-thought-of treatments) and make much faster recoveries. I can dream. If even one patient is diagnosed earlier and recovers faster, writing this book will have been worth the struggle.

One of my fondest memories of success was watching a patient who was ill for many years with CFS embrace the concept of pacing and exercising using the 10 percent rule. The patient changed his diet accordingly (see chapter 4). The patient was able to set up better boundaries with his family to safeguard the successes made. The patient went on to add the muscle strengthening exercises correctly. The patient had been ill, quite severely (energy was 3 out of 10 initially), for more than ten years. He was able to go back to work and successfully work part-time for four hours five days a week when in his late fifties. This happened over a number of years. Amazing!

I had another patient with severe fibromyalgia pain that kept the patient bed confined for a number of years. By helping the patient deal with the pain and anxiety, and teaching her to eat more nutritionally, she was able to mobilize slowly. She went from being confined to her bedroom and the upstairs of her house to eventually going downstairs. The next step was slowly using a walker and then a cane. This person has now become an artist and creates special paintings that delight all that are fortunate enough to obtain one.

The Functional Capacity Scale is a guide. It is not perfect, and sometimes patients have significant differences between physical and cognitive function. If a person is better physically than they are cognitively—for example, if they are at a 5 and have 50 percent energy and can walk ten to twenty minutes a day, but cognitively they still have difficulty concentrating—I would have them use the lower score, which would be 4/10. Many patients improve both physically and cognitively together. However, some improve cognitively first and then physically, while others progress in the opposite way. In my practice I find that most progress over time.

ENERGY CONSERVATION

There are certain guidelines to learn about energy conservation. You can spend your energy in three different ways: emotionally, mentally, or physically. You can only spend your energy once. If you have had a fight with your kids, you may not be able to pay the bills because you have already spent your energy quota for the day emotionally with your kids. Not that you should avoid your kids, but there might be better ways of handling them instead of getting angry with them. The entire family is affected by this illness, so everyone must participate in order to make the home situation run as smoothly as possible. You might need outside counseling to work through dealing with the impact of a chronic illness and to build a more workable family situation where the everyday workload is evenly distributed. In other words, if you used to "do it all" for your family, you will have to delegate some of your responsibilities in order for everyday things such as preparing dinner to be accomplished. When you pace yourself, you are learning the principles of physical energy conservation.

What Your Doctor Can Do for You

Your doctor can help you with energy conservation by filling out a disability parking permit, which allows you to park in a disability parking space. You *are* disabled, because on a bad day you cannot walk very far. These parking spaces will give you access to the nearest entrance of the store where you will be shopping. This allows you to get out of your house more frequently for shopping and at the same time conserve energy so that you can actually do the shopping in a focused way instead of using your energy walking to and from your car in the parking lot. I know from my patients that this is a really gut-wrenching issue. It forces those with more severe forms of CFS/FM to confront the fact that they are disabled.

Again, I tell my patients to "park their pride at home" and pick it back up when they return. If patients do use the disability parking permit, it gives them much more freedom to get out more frequently and remain connected to the outside world. It helps them to conserve their energy and do what needs to be done as opposed to wasting it walking to and from the store. I encourage my patients to be as active as they can be without crashing. If patients remain at home alone they often become very isolated and can develop anxieties to the point of panic attacks when going back out into the world outside their home. Patients need to be as active as possible to stay emotionally healthy and also to prevent osteoporosis in the long-term. Those patients who are bedridden cannot drive.

Self Care or Bathing

If a person is too tired to give themselves a bath at least once a week, they should be assessed by the local visiting nurse or home-makers association. In Toronto this service is provided for by the CCAC which stands for Community Care Access Centres. This service provides personal care for people who cannot bathe themselves because they are too unsteady to get in and of out the bathtub unassisted and may fall or injure themselves. It may also provide a couple of hours of homemaking services. When a person is at an energy level of 1, they really do need ongoing support by other family members. Unfortunately the only long-term care facilities that can care for people at this low energy level until they recover sufficiently are nursing homes or residential facilities. Not a great choice for younger people. CFS/FM are poorly understood conditions, and none of the agencies that I am familiar with provide these services. The need is certainly there for this kind of care; however, most often it gets left to friends or family of the patient. This is always true when children are ill with CFS/FM. A residential facility similar to a cancer or HIV-AIDS hospice would be ideal and would help patients at this low level of functioning to begin to recover. I continue to dream.

Energy Conservation—Some Examples

Bathing/Self Care

In terms of general principles, energy conservation means doing things in such a way as to reduce the amount of energy output needed. Consider, for example, bathing. It is something we all must do. People with CFS are exhausted and FM patients are in pain, both of which can interfere with this task that most healthy people take for granted. A way to reduce energy while bathing is to sit down on a shower chair in the shower as opposed to standing up and showering or getting stuck in the tub without the upper body strength to get yourself out. I find it very helpful to have patients assessed by an occupational therapist. These therapists actually go into patients' homes and look at their individual situation to determine if the patient can be helped during bathing by installing, for example, grab bars in the bathroom or by using a shower chair. Be sure that the chair is stable. They usually have rubber feet on the bottom so they don't slide around in the bathtub. I find it helps when you put a small towel on the back of the plastic chair so that it is not cold when you lean back against it, which might cause your muscles to cramp and hurt more. It also helps to install a raised toilet seat so that you can get up off the toilet more easily when your leg muscles are weak. If you are too fatigued to walk to the bathroom, then a bedside commode is helpful.

When you have your menstrual cycle and need a wash but are just too tired to have a bath, consider using a bidet if you have one or using a perineal bottle. A perineal bottle is a clear bottle that you fill up with warm water and spray the water over your private parts or your perineum after you clean yourself with toilet paper. You can often buy these at a pharmacy or drug store if you ask the druggist for it. If it is not available any small empty squeeze bottle (e.g., an empty liquid dishwashing soap bottle) filled with warm water will work. You can also use this to keep yourself clean on other days when you are just too tired to take a shower or bath.

Another example of energy conservation is reducing the energy used to dry your hair. Instead of standing up and holding the blow-dryer over your head in one hand and brushing your hair with the other hand, try this: Lie or sit down with your head in one of those old-fashioned bag type hair dryers that slip over your hair. That way you can be resting and drying your hair at the same time. When I had meningitis I did this because I was just too physically tired to raise my hands over my head and blow my hair dry. Another method is to place your handheld blow-dryer in its stand and position it on the counter facing you. Then sit on a chair in front of the counter so that you can literally sit down and have the blow dryer directed at your hair instead of trying to hold it above your head. Any time you have to hold your hands above your head it is very tiring, so avoid it.

Cooking

In the kitchen, an example of energy conservation is sitting down to cook on a stool rather than standing up. Instead of trying to cook intricate meals, try and keep it simple by using one-pot meals either in a roasting pan in the oven using low heat, or using a crock-pot. Make a double batch of a main course and freeze the other half for another day when you cannot cook. Another example would be to buy fresh or frozen vegetables that are already chopped and washed. Frozen are often better because they do not start to go moldy when you don't eat them up in a few days. Start making dinner in the morning or when your level of energy is the best and break it up into little steps. During the preparation, plan a rest period after each step. For example, wash the lettuce for a salad, rest; mix up the various ingredients needed to make a meatloaf, rest; finally chop the vegetables, and rest. When you need to wash the dishes, put them in soapy water to soak. They will almost wash themselves. After you have washed them leave them on a drying rack to dry. When your pots are clean leave them clean on the stove so that you do not have to bend over in the cupboard to find them next time. Conserve your energy.

Cleaning

If possible, get help with the vacuuming, floors, and bathroom. Lower your standards. You cannot keep the immaculate house you had in the past. Aim for clean enough. The more fatigued you are the more cluttered your home will be. Try to break tasks down into fifteen-minute segments so that they don't seem so overwhelming.

Bills

Try to put important bills and papers in one special spot each time so that when you have the energy to go through them you know where they are and you do not have to search for them. Also, consolidate your bills and do as much over the phone or on-line paying of bills as possible. If this is not possible, try to arrange to have your bills paid through your bank account on a regular basis, like your car insurance and house payments. If you need help, try to get a family member or friend you trust to help you with this. Often simple things like writing a check or balancing a checkbook can seem like a huge mountain to climb for many patients.

Shopping

If you do have energy to walk for a few minutes but find grocery shopping too incapacitating, try to go to a larger grocery store; often they will have scooters that you can sit on to buy the few things that you need. If you have access to a grocery service that provides on-line ordering services and delivers, that is even better. Here in Toronto, several large chain grocery stores deliver, which is extremely helpful for disabled people. There is often a small fee for this, but it is worth every penny in terms of conserving your energy so you don't crash after you grocery shop. Also if you do shop, always use a cart you can lean on. This will help with your balance and will support you if your upper body strength is reduced.

If your energy is slightly higher, you will probably find it useful to use a walker. This especially applies to people who are starting to walk about five minutes outside the home. By having a walker—especially with a seat—you can walk for a few minutes and then sit down.

When people are to the point of being able to get out and get their groceries and actually walk, getting stuck in line in the grocery store can lead to physical fatigue, feeling faint, or actually fainting. I advise patients to carry a lightweight cane with three legs with a small collapsible seat attached. The handle of the cane can be hooked over the handle of the shopping cart. If patients feel very fatigued waiting in line, they can open the cane chair out and sit while they wait. Some patients bring a small collapsible lightweight camp seat for use when traveling outside the home for the same reason.

If you do suddenly feel dizzy or faint and you are out somewhere, it is better to immediately lie down flat on the floor. This will help you to feel better, even though you will no doubt feel embarrassed. This helps to bring the blood that has pooled in your legs while you were standing back to your head and prevent a faint or black-out. It is better to consciously lie down than to fall down and end up in the ER for stitches because you split your head open when you hit the floor. Of course, after you finish reading this book you will be pacing so well that this will not happen to you.

Socializing

Patients should continue to socialize as their energy permits. CFS/FM are very socially isolating illnesses, and as a result patients can feel very lonely. Socializing can take many forms. It can be as simple as a phone call or it may involve going out to visit at someone else's house. In both cases you need to keep within your energy boundaries. When you are on the phone it helps to set a timer and tell the person that you only have a few minutes to chat with them. At first this will be difficult. But when you see the results of not crashing it will get easier.

There may be times when you are too fatigued to talk on the phone. If that is the case, do not answer the phone—either use your answering machine or take the phone off the hook. Put yourself first. Say no to toxic people who drain you and waste your time and energy listening to them.

If you want to visit, ask your host ahead of time if there is a bedroom that you can lie down in while you rest during your visit. You need to keep the same schedule when you are visiting as when you are at home. You will be surprised at people's reactions. Most of my patients tell me that their friends were so glad that they could come for a visit that needing a time to rest was not a problem. If you want to keep your friends, you have to spend some time with them in such a way that you do not crash. One of my patients goes to visit a friend by lying on her friend's couch while her friend does the laundry, etc. Her friend spends her breaks with the patient and the patient rests while her friend works around the house. Both the patient and her friend get what they need without anyone being a burden to the other—a win-win situation.

Holiday Celebrations—Birthdays, Thanksgiving, etc.
I break down all holidays into five categories: food, people, presents, spiritual celebration, and place. Religious holidays like Christmas are always the busiest because people often have such high expectations of themselves and others.

So when they are planning for a holiday, I ask patients questions to help them figure out how best to celebrate without crashing. I ask them first, "What is the one thing that means the most to you?" For example, at Christmas, it might be the meal with family and friends, the visiting with family and friends, the presents, the decorating of the Christmas tree, or going to church. Each patient has different answers. I ask them next, "What is the *one* thing that *you want* to do most?"

They pick one thing. Then we discuss how they can do that *one* thing. For example one patient really liked having the Christmas meal at her house. She used to love to decorate the house, the tree, and make a delicious meal for her family. So instead she got her friends and family together weeks before Christmas and watched them decorate the house and tree while she sat on the couch and watched. She still got her house decorated and she enjoyed watching them do it. She was too exhausted to cook, so everyone in her family brought a dish. She bought festive paper plates and napkins. They had a lovely dinner, which she enjoyed, and she didn't crash in bed for days afterward like she had the previous year.

Other patients go to a restaurant or order a full Christmas meal including the dressing from a nearby restaurant. This satisfies their need to have a good visit with their extended family. Try it; you'll see that learning how not to crash is worth it.

When it comes to presents and you have young children, get to know your favorite catalogs. When I had meningitis, I asked my kids to circle the presents that they wanted Santa to bring them. When it got close to Christmas I asked them to tell me the one present they liked the best, because after all Santa could only carry so many toys in his sack. They picked it and I ordered it. I liked the process so much that I did it for many years after that.

If you have older kids, consider gift cards or just good old cash. If you cannot afford to continue to buy gifts because your finances have greatly decreased as a result of being ill, then consider not buying gifts this year. Start some new traditions based on your new situation. If you still want to continue with gift giving, consider having a draw and buying for only one member of the family instead of for everyone. This obviously needs to be discussed in advance of the holiday.

If you are too tired to go to church, other alternatives are watching church on TV, going to an earlier service (instead of the midnight service) or asking someone from your church to come and visit you during the holiday season. Don't be afraid to sit while others are standing if you are too tired. Some of my patients even bring a collapsible lawn chair or chaise lounge and leave it at church so they can keep their legs elevated. If your church pews are wide enough, you could even lie down during the service—some of my patients do this. If you plan on this, make sure that you tell the people around you and your priest or minister so that they do not become alarmed when they see you lying down during the service.

Energy Conservation—Summary
Depending on your energy/pain levels, the above-mentioned examples may or may not apply to you. The point is to show you a few of the potentially hundreds of situations or ways in which you can personally conserve energy. Pacing and energy conservation will always be a work in progress and evolve through the course of your illness. These are some examples to guide you and get you started on the road to recovery. Energy conservation—master it and begin your recovery process. Remember that setbacks are part of the process; accept them and appreciate the overall gains. Don't fall into the trap of comparing your health with your pre-illness life. This is not constructive, it is *destructive* to your mental health and keeps you stuck in the past. You need to measure your recovery by what you were like when you were first ill and at your worst. By doing this, you will see just how far you have really come on your road to recovery and see the slow and steady progress you have made by learning how to practice pacing and energy conservation.

For more tips on energy conservation, please see the Appendix for "Energy Conservation: Achieving a Balance of Work, Rest and Play" by Carson et al.

SLEEP HYGIENE

Restoring sleep is essential for improving your health. You need to do everything possible to encourage your body to get the best sleep it can every single night. Sleep hygiene doesn't mean taking a shower and washing up before bed, it refers to the ways and means of maximizing your sleep. It is a whole menu of individual items that promote a restful sleep, and it is a critical part of the recovery process in CFS/FM. Improving sleep, even a little, can make a tremendous difference to a patient's symptom reduction and quality of life. Sleep is an important part of any energy conservation/pacing program because it is the time when replenishment of your energy battery takes place. Many physiological processes are hard at work during deep sleep, including immune regulation and repair or detoxification processes.

Here are some general sleep hygiene principles for improving sleep. Other means such as medications, herbals, relaxation techniques, etc. will be discussed as we proceed through the chapters.

- Your bedroom should be as dark as possible for maximum melatonin release. Use blackout curtains, blinds, or a sleeping mask.
- Your bedroom should be used for sleeping only. Remove the television and computer if possible.
- The bedroom environment should be quiet and free of clutter. It should be an oasis from the rest of the world.
- The bedroom should be warm and comfortable but not too hot.
- Keep a regular schedule; go to bed at the same time every night, even on weekends.
- Avoid crashing, because if you crash you will be too exhausted to fall asleep and your brain will be over-stimulated and difficult to turn off for sleep.
- Eliminate caffeine-containing beverages and food. These stimulate you and keep you awake.
- Some patients require daytime naps. After lunch is OK, but don't take a nap after dinner.

- Try to get some physical activity/exercise daily as this helps to tire you out. However, avoid exercise just before bedtime as it is often stimulating.
- Avoid eating meals late at night.
- Use relaxation techniques (like meditation, described later) in the evening.
- Invest in a comfortable mattress. Use an egg crate or soft foam to cover your mattress if it is too hard for you.
- For noise problems, earplugs (silicone works best) or sound-proofing may help some, while others respond to steady sounds (e.g., white noise devices).
- Avoid TV news and action movies before bed; they can increase anxiety and worry.
- If your partner wakes you up every morning when getting ready for work and you have the space, consider sleeping in different bedrooms. Sleep is right up there with food and water as a requirement for good health.

CHAPTER SUMMARY

- CFS/FM patients need to approach day-to-day life in a new way, one that includes advance planning.
- Pacing is central to recovery efforts. After recognition of new activity limitations true progress can begin.
- The activity log and functional capacity scale are your educational tools and allow for identification of physical/mental stressors and their role in symptom expression.
- Set short-term goals in gradually increasing daily activities.
- Utilize those around you and government/private institutions for assistance.
- While gradually increasing activity, always consider the principles of energy conservation so that you have energy for the things that you enjoy.
- Accept that setbacks may occur; they are part of the recovery process.
- Work through emotional scars left by your chronic illness.

- Sleep is essential; remember to follow the guidelines of sleep hygiene.
- Learn to say no.
- Compare your illness state now with CFS/FM onset, not your pre-illness life.
- Remain optimistic and hopeful. It is a slow road to recovery with twists and turns, but progression is possible.

CHAPTER FOUR

NUTRITIONAL SUPPORT

FOOD AS MEDICINE

We have all heard the saying "You are what you eat." However, it may be more appropriate to say that you are what the plants and animals you eat ate! Both plant and animal food processing has changed dramatically in the last hundred years. Numerous chemicals have been introduced into the food supply in the form of food dyes, preservatives, flavor enhancers, and pesticides. Canadian and U.S. research indicates that the fruits and vegetables in today's produce section contain lower amounts of certain vitamins and minerals compared with twenty years ago, most likely a result of soil nutrient depletion. Animal rearing practices now involve the feeding of grains (mostly corn) and the administration of growth hormone and multiple antibiotics. In addition, high-fat, chemical-laden, sugary snack foods are everywhere—it's a challenge to avoid them. What's worse is that

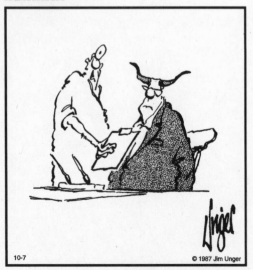

HERMAN®

10-7   © 1987 Jim Unger

**"Have you heard that expression,
'You are what you eat?'"**

CFS and FM patients are often sensitive to or intolerant of the ingredients and chemicals that are in processed food, yet they are understandably drawn to convenience foods when tired or in pain.

The whole situation seems overwhelming, but it doesn't have to be. There are easy-to-follow steps for the CFS/FM patient on the road to healthy nutrition. Basic dietary advice for CFS/FM patients is not too different from that for all North Americans or that used to treat and prevent cardiovascular disease or type II diabetes. Recent research suggests that food/chemical intolerances may be playing a role in both CFS and FM and that addressing these may improve symptoms. Additional considerations for those with known or suspected food intolerances will be made.

It can be difficult to eat healthily when quick and easy "meals" (I'll use that term loosely!) in the form of frozen dinners and fast food are readily available. When the pain of FM or the fatigue in CFS is particularly bad, it is understandable that a frozen dinner or a fast food option may seem attractive—however, no one, healthy or otherwise, should be making these choices a regular part of their diet. The vast majority of fast foods are high in saturated and trans fats, simple carbohydrates (those without fiber) and are devoid of important vitamins, minerals, and plant nutrients called phytochemicals. In short, the standard American diet (SAD) provides plenty of calories but not enough nutrients. Inappropriate dietary choices have been linked to a number of chronic illnesses in modern society, most notably cardiovascular disease, diabetes, cancer, and the new epidemic of obesity.

Despite the pain and fatigue, it is critically important in recovery efforts to make healthy choices. If you are fortunate enough to have someone to help prepare food, then enlist their help. As high-functioning individuals pre-illness, it is often hard for CFS/FM patients to bring themselves to ask for assistance. As Dr. Bested previously discussed, learning to delegate and use the help of others (in the kitchen and beyond) is extremely important.

Table 1. The ten fruits and ten vegetables (non-organic) with the lowest pesticide ratings.

1) Pineapples	1) Avocado
2) Plantains	2) Cauliflower
3) Mangoes	3) Brussels sprouts
4) Bananas	4) Asparagus
5) Watermelon	5) Radishes
6) Plums	6) Broccoli
7) Kiwi Fruit	7) Onions
8) Blueberries	8) Okra
9) Papaya	9) Cabbage
10) Grapefruit	10) Eggplant

Table 2. The twelve non-organic fruits and vegetables (in order) with the highest concentration of pesticides.

1) Strawberries	7) Celery
2) Bell peppers (tie with spinach)	8) Apples
	9) Apricots
3) Spinach	10) Green beans
4) Cherries (USA)	11) Grapes
5) Peaches	12) Cucumbers (Chilean)
6) Cantaloupe (Mexico)	

Before examining special CFS/FM diets, it is essential to first lay down the basic healthy eating framework. A number of years ago, the U.S. National Cancer Institute launched the "5 a Day for Better Health" program with the goal of increasing public awareness and providing information on the value of dietary fruits and vegetables. Eating a minimum of five servings of fruits and vegetables is probably the most significant step a person can take in healthy nutrition. Sadly, while statistics may show the average North American adult is close to the five servings, there are four "vegetables" that account for over half of total intake—tomato (mostly as processed sauce/ketchup), iceberg lettuce, potato (mostly fried), and onion. Orange juice accounts for a large percentage of total fruit intake. It seems clear that the big problem is lack of variety. A diet devoid of a mixture of fruits and vegetables will result in a decreased intake of the more than twenty-five thousand different phytochemicals, which are critical to the antioxidant defenses in CFS/FM. While a lowered nutrient value in today's fruits and vegetables may be an issue worthy of further research, the limited data is not cause for alarm; if anything, it's just one more reason to increase your daily intake. Also, in an effort to lower the chemical load and perhaps get more nutritious fruits and vegetables, CFS/FM patients should seek out organic produce. However, organic choices can be very expensive, and certain non-organic produce really doesn't differ too much from organic in terms of pesticide use.

Avoiding the twelve most contaminated fruits and vegetables in non-organic produce can reduce an individual's health risks from pesticides on foods by 50 percent. (Environmental Working Group, compiled from FDA and EPA data. For more information, see www.ewg.org.)

PHYTOCHEMICALS AND HEALTH PROMOTION

I've mentioned phytochemicals a couple of times, so let's define what they are and why they are so important in CFS/FM. Phytochemicals are plant-based substances that give plants the color, texture, and taste that we experience. Plants, for their own survival and health, manufacture phytochemicals; it is not surprising, then, that they are of value in human health. In contrast to vitamins and minerals, phytochemicals are not considered "essential" for the maintenance of life. However, the value of phytochemicals in health promotion and disease prevention is becoming increasingly clear. In the human body, phytochemicals act as potent antioxidants, stimulate the immune system, regulate cholesterol, and modulate enzymatic activity and hormone metabolism. In addition, phytochemicals have anti-inflammatory, antiviral, and antibacterial activities. Studies have shown that phytochemicals can help to prevent cancer and cardiovascular disease and, importantly for those with CFS/FM, have the ability to protect the nervous system.

One of the largest and best-known groups of phytochemicals is the polyphenol class—more than eight thousand polyphenolic structures are currently known. Within the polyphenolic family are the flavonoids, a group with numerous scientific studies attesting to their health-promoting properties. Flavonoids include flavones, flavonols, flavanones, catechins, anthocyanins, and isoflavones. To ensure consumption of different types of flavonoids, a variety of fruits and vegetables must be consumed. For example, the catechins are found in high amounts in tea; the anthocyanins in blueberries, cherries, and elderberry; the isoflavones in soy; flavonols in apples; and so on.

Another class of phytochemicals are the carotenoids, which include beta-carotene, lutein, lycopene, and zeaxanthin. All have documented antioxidant and other health-promoting activity. Beta-carotene is found in carrots and other orange vegetables, lutein in dark greens such as broccoli and kale, lycopene in red veggies such as red peppers and tomatoes, and zeaxanthin in yellow and green vegetables such as corn and spinach. In addition, there are other beneficial phytochemicals such as limonene in citrus fruits, ellagic acid in berries, and sulphoraphane in Brussels sprouts, kale, cabbage, and broccoli. In order to get the most out of phytochemicals, CFS/FM patients require the entire color spectrum of fruits and vegetables—variety is the key.

THE SYNERGY OF PHYTOCHEMICALS

The research demonstrating the value of fruits and vegetables in the diet has led to immense additional research on phytochemicals. Until recently, the focus of research related to plant chemicals has been on isolated forms—for example, the study of isolated beta-carotene or the vitamins in plant foods such as vitamins C and E. The study of isolated antioxidant vitamins in human health has yielded mixed findings; the results are not as strong as those involving the whole plant with its supporting cast of phytochemicals. Antioxidants act in synergy, much like an orchestra, and research is beginning to show the benefits of taking antioxidants together. For example, isoflavones have increased antioxidant activity in the presence of vitamin C, and the antioxidant activity of both alfalfa extract and isolated isoflavones has been shown to dramatically increase antioxidant activity in the presence of Acerola cherry extract. In fact, research shows that two antioxidants together have greater antioxidant potential than the sum of the two individually. Many researchers are now beginning to look at how whole food extracts and herbal extracts work together.

Although best known as antioxidants, phytochemical promotion of health does not solely reside in antioxidant activity. In the case of blueberry extract, there are neuroprotective properties that appear to be the result of both antioxidant activity and other, yet-to-be-determined, pathways. There is still much to be learned about the specific ways in which phytochemicals positively influence health.

As discussed by Dr. Bested, there is a growing body of research showing that CFS/FM are disorders not only with increased oxidative stress but also diminished antioxidant capacity. In plain English, CFS/FM patients really need to boost their dietary antioxidant intake to support recovery efforts. The best way to increase antioxidant status is to increase your intake of fruits and vegetables. Supplements can provide additional help, and I'll discuss them later, but they are not a substitute for a colorful diet. There are volumes of international research on the health benefits of *dietary* vitamins, minerals, and phytochemicals, but as mentioned, when scientists isolate a single nutrient or plant chemical and research it, the results are often disappointing. There are lots of studies that support diet over supplements; one recent example with Alzheimer's disease provides a clear example. Oxidative stress and free radical formation are thought to play a role in the development of Alzheimer's, so researchers have been examining diet and supplements to assess their influence on the illness. Two separate studies in the *Journal of the American Medical Association* in 2002 found that foods rich in antioxidant vitamins C and E can reduce the risk of developing Alzheimer's, while vitamins C and E in supplement form were of no value. Bottom line—while there may be benefits to taking select supplements, spend your money on *food* first because it really is strong medicine.

Functional foods are relatively new products appearing in health food stores and supermarkets: examples include powdered whole fruit and vegetable extracts with only the water removed. These are somewhat different than isolated vitamin/mineral supplements, and quality functional foods may be valuable for CFS/FM patients as a means of supplementing a healthy diet and conserving energy. In fact, new research on one such powdered food supplement, greens+, showed it can improve energy and

Table 3. A variety of fruits: When was the last time you had some of these fruits?

Red Apples	Grapefruits	Brown Pears
Blood Oranges	Golden Kiwis	Avocados
Cherries	Lemons	Green Apples
Cranberries	Mangoes	Green Grapes
Red Grapes	Nectarines	Honeydews
Pink Grapefruit	Oranges	Kiwifruits
Red Grapefruit	Papayas	Limes
Red Pears	Peaches	Green Pears
Pomegranates	Yellow Pears	Blackberries
Raspberries	Persimmons	Blueberries
Strawberries	Tangerines	Black Currants
Watermelon	Yellow Watermelons	Plums
Yellow Apples	Bananas	Elderberries
Apricots	Dates	Purple Figs
Cantaloupes	White Nectarines	Purple Grapes
Yellow Figs	White Peaches	Raisins

vitality in healthy adults. I will discuss this in more detail in the supplements chapter.

PROTEIN, CARBOHYDRATES, AND FATS

Now that you are consuming at least five servings of fruits and veggies a day, we can turn our attention to the other important components of a healthy meal. There are no simple answers, but as the research pours in it seems that the EatWise Food Pyramid, developed at Harvard Medical School (shown on the next page), provides the most appropriate advice. As you can see, the emphasis is on a staple of whole grains, the carbohydrates that are rich in dietary fiber. This is particularly important in CFS/FM because carbohydrates that are devoid of fiber (refined cereals, white bread, plain pasta) can cause a rapid rise in blood sugar and spike

Table 4. A Variety of veggies: When was the last time you had some of these vegetables?

Beets	Cauliflower	Green Beans
Red Peppers	Garlic	Green Cabbage
Radishes	Ginger	Chayote Squash
Radicchio	Jicama	Cucumbers
Red Onions	Mushrooms	Endive
Red Potatoes	Onions	Leeks
Rhubarb	Parsnips	Dark Green Lettuce
Tomatoes	White Potatoes	Green Onions
Yellow Beets	Shallots	Okra
Butternut Squash	Turnips	Peas
Carrots	Artichokes	Green Peppers
Yellow Peppers	Arugula	Snow Peas
Yellow Potatoes	Asparagus	Spinach
Pumpkins	Bok Choy	Snap Peas
Rutabagas	Broccoli	Zucchini
Yellow Squash	Broccoli Rabe	Eggplant
Sweet Corn	Brussels Sprouts	Purple Potatoes
Sweet Potatoes	Chinese Cabbage	

insulin levels. Insulin is released to handle the blood sugar, and the end result is a quick drop in blood sugar shortly thereafter; for many CFS/FM patients, the symptoms of hypoglycemia kick in. Symptoms of hypoglycemia include fatigue, anxiety, cognitive difficulties, dizziness, and nausea—experiences that are already all too familiar to CFS/FM patients. Someone who has CFS/FM cannot afford to get into this vicious cycle of quick rises and falls in blood glucose. Balancing blood sugar is extremely important in symptom management, so follow Harvard's advice and choose unrefined cereals and whole grain breads and pasta as well as brown rice.

The Harvard EatWise Pyramid encourages liberal consumption of deeply colored fruits and vegetables and also places more emphasis on healthy oils such as olive and canola oils—there is a clear distinction between types of fat. This is important because government and dietetic groups have instilled a fear of dietary fat

Figure 1. The EatWise Food Pyramid.

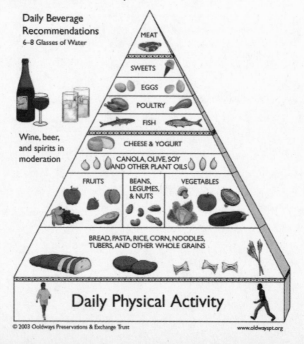

Daily Beverage Recommendations
6–8 Glasses of Water

MEAT

SWEETS

EGGS

POULTRY

FISH

CHEESE & YOGURT

CANOLA, OLIVE, SOY AND OTHER PLANT OILS

FRUITS

BEANS, LEGUMES, & NUTS

VEGETABLES

Wine, beer, and spirits in moderation

BREAD, PASTA, RICE, CORN, NOODLES, TUBERS, AND OTHER WHOLE GRAINS

Daily Physical Activity

into North Americans whithout the recognition that there are oils that promote health, whereas saturated and trans fats have a negative influence on health. In addition, there is greater emphasis on healthy protein choices such as cheese and yogurt, seafood, poultry, and eggs—while red meat is relegated to the pyramid tip. Harvard researchers recommend one to two servings of dairy a day (or a calcium supplement), and a multivitamin for most adults is suggested—a cheap nutritional insurance policy. Preliminary research by the experts from Harvard Medical School indicates that an individual who eats according to the new pyramid will be at a lower risk of major chronic disease.

ESSENTIAL FATS

For the last twenty years or so, fats have gotten a bad name. Yes, saturated fat and artificially hardened fats (trans fats) are harmful, and for the CFS/FM patient, they may contribute to the production of inflammatory chemicals in the body. But there are good fats too. Certain fats can have many positive effects for the patient with CFS/FM. Let's take a close look at the type of fat that a CFS/FM patient should focus on, omega-3 fatty acids. Omega-3 fatty acids and omega-6 fatty acids are considered essential for life, and we need to take them in from dietary sources because we can't manufacture them on our own; hence the name essential fatty acids (EFA). We can, however, make changes to EFA once they are consumed, and these changes are critical to the CFS/FM patient. Fatty acid intake influences important body chemicals called prostaglandins and cytokines, and fatty acids also influence the makeup of nerve cells—all of which can affect CFS/FM symptoms.

Omega-3 fatty acids are fats that are found in abundance in many types of seafood. They are also found in high amounts in flax seeds, walnuts, and canola oil, and to a lesser degree in soy oil, wild game meats, and green vegetables. The omega-6 fatty acid is everywhere in a typical Western diet (corn, sunflower, sesame, and safflower oils are examples). Not that these oils are particularly bad, but they are being over-consumed in relation to omega-3 fats. The ratio of omega-6 to omega-3 fats in the Western diet has been drastically altered; it is estimated that North Americans consume only 20 percent of the omega-3 fatty acids today that they consumed a hundred years ago. Throughout human evolution, the ratio of omega-6 to omega-3 intake was close to 1:1, but, incredibly, in today's Western diet it approaches 20:1! While omega-6 fatty acids are important, their over-consumption is linked to inflammation and a number of chronic illnesses. A panel of thirty of the world's leading essential fatty acid experts has stated that the ideal ratio in the promotion of health is close to 1:1, omega-6 to omega-3. This recommended ratio was published in the *Journal of the American College of Nutrition* in 1999, making it very clear that omega-6 supplementation is unnecessary. Some groups in the food industry have caught on, producing omega-3–enriched eggs, but in general change has been slow. CFS/FM patients need desperately to ensure they are getting plenty of omega-3 fatty acids and at the same time reducing intake of the previously mentioned omega-6 oils. Once again, supplements are available (these will be discussed later), but dietary choices should be prioritized. Consider cooking with canola oil and including ground flax seeds in your diet.

Research shows that omega-3 fats not only protect against cardiovascular disease but may also be beneficial in CFS and FM, inflammatory disorders, gastrointestinal disorders, skin conditions, depression, diabetes, weight control, menstrual cramps, and prevention of preterm deliveries in pregnancy. The list of conditions that fish oil may benefit seems overwhelming, and many of the trials of fish oils have been performed by leading university-based scientists and published in very prestigious medical journals.

SPECIAL DIETS

So we have the basics down. You are now consuming a diet rich in fruits, vegetables, essential fats, and whole grains—shouldn't this be the end of the nutrition chapter? Sadly, many CFS/FM

Table 5. Various sources of EPA and DHA.

Fish/Seafood	Total EPA/DHA (mg/100g)
Mackerel	2300
Chinook salmon	1900
Herring	1700
Anchovy	1400
Sardine	1400
Coho salmon	1200
Trout	600
Spiny lobster	500
Halibut	400
Shrimp	300
Catfish	300
Sole	200
Cod	200

Table 6. Omega-6 and omega-3 content (%) of dietary oils.

Oil	Omega-6	Omega-3
Safflower	75	0
Sunflower	65	0
Corn	54	0
Cottonseed	50	0
Sesame	42	0
Peanut	32	0
Soybean	51	7
Canola	20	9
Walnut	52	10
Flax	14	57

patients seem to develop intolerances to certain foods after they become ill. Food intolerances must be distinguished from food allergies, a more readily diagnosable condition where there is a fairly immediate reaction to (for example) shellfish, peanuts, or bee products. Food intolerances are usually slower to manifest, with more vague symptoms such as gastrointestinal complaints, headaches, fatigue, joint pain, or cognitive difficulties. For some patients the intolerant food is easy to recognize, and they eliminate it with success. But for others with numerous intolerances it can be a little tricky.

To make matters worse, there is no well-established blood test to determine food intolerances. Lack of a good laboratory test has led a large number of physicians to suggest that food intolerances are merely somatic complaints (physical complaints of psychological origin)—basically, it's all in your head. Patients with chronic illnesses who report food intolerances have often been dismissed as having a psychiatric illness or as merely manifesting "somatization traits," the medical term for converting mental experiences into vague bodily symptoms. Recent research has shown, however, that not only can food intolerances cause a defined physiological response, but that this response can indeed involve the immune system.

Patients with CFS/FM often report new or increased sensitivity to noise, light, odors, chemicals, and foods after the onset of illness. Many patients make attempts to limit exposure to these aggravating factors in an effort to reduce symptoms. Two studies presented at the American Association for Chronic Fatigue Syndrome International Scientific Conference in Seattle in 2001 indicate that dietary modifications may play a positive role in symptom management. The first study, presented by Nisenbaum et al., showed that 54 percent of CFS patients (sample from Kansas) attempt dietary changes, and of these individuals, 73 percent reported that dietary changes were beneficial in reducing fatigue. Dietary changes were reported as more beneficial than vitamins, herbal remedies, and exercise. It was unspecified whether these improvements were thought to be due to the addition or the elimination of certain foods. In the second study, this one presented by Australian researchers, CFS patients eliminated wheat, milk, benzoates, nitrites, nitrates, food colorings, and other additives from their diet. Of the CFS patients who complied (50 percent), the results were impressive: 90 percent reported improvement in the severity of symptoms across multiple body systems, with significant reduction in fatigue, recurrent fever, sore throat, muscle pain, headache, joint pain, and cognitive dysfunction. In addition, the elimination protocol resulted in a marked improvement in irritable bowel–like symptoms.

In our own research, presented at the Sixth International Conference on CFS, FM, and Related Illnesses, held in Washington, D.C., in February 2003, Dr. Bested and I found that 88 percent of CFS patients (a sample from metro Toronto) attempt dietary modifications in an effort to manage CFS symptoms. Of the patients who made changes to their diets, 73 percent reported that these efforts were helpful to some degree. In addition, we found that over half of CFS patients report food sensitivities after the onset of illness. Most commonly, patients report sensitivities to wheat, dairy, corn, tomato, and caffeinated beverages. Symptoms associated with food intolerances were most often fatigue, gas/bloating, headaches, diarrhea, nausea, and pain.

The findings reported at these international scientific conferences are supported by earlier publications by Borok in the *South African Medical Journal* (1989) and Gibson in the *Journal of Nutritional and Environmental Medicine* (1999). Borok reported significant improvement among twenty CFS patients after removing certain foods from their diet, with milk, wheat, and corn among the top offenders. In Gibson's report a wheat-free diet was used along with nutritional supplementation and homeopathy, and after four months 70 percent of the sixty-four CFS patients showed improvement in physical symptoms and mental outlook.

The elimination and rechallenge of foods and additives is also an emerging area of research in FM. Researchers from the Thomas Jefferson University Hospital recently reported the results of a study that involved the elimination and rechallenge of certain foods. The results, published in the *Journal of the American College of Clinical Nutrition* (2001), showed that half of the seventeen FM patients had a significant reduction in pain during the elimination phase, while 76 percent reported a reduction in fatigue, headaches, and gastrointestinal symptoms. These same symptoms were made worse during the challenge phase—in this case, corn, wheat, dairy, citrus, and refined sugar were among the top offending foods. Food additives may also aggravate the symptoms of FM. In a series of case studies published in the *Annals of Pharmacotherapy* (2001), the removal of dietary monosodium glutamate (MSG) and aspartame (in most diet soft drinks and chewing gum) led to major improvement in symptoms and rechallenge caused a marked aggravation of symptoms. CFS/FM patients should avoid both regular and aspartame-containing diet soda. A number of companies are now using sucralose as a sugar substitute in sugar-free gums and soda; this may be a good, more tolerable alternative if you can't break the habit!

The question remains, might all of these studies showing some improvement in CFS/FM after dietary changes merely represent a "placebo" effect, one that is medicating a somatization trait? In simple terms, it's all in your mind. Thankfully, recent research published in the prestigious journal *Lancet* has not only validated the symptoms of those with food intolerance but has also demonstrated a physiological mechanism and challenged the false assumption of the presence of a psychiatric disorder. In the study by Jacobsen et al. (2000), patients with perceived food intolerance were asked to consume foods they had previously eliminated. The patients had normal routine laboratory tests and no lactase deficiency. After consuming milk and wheat for two weeks, those with food intolerance were found to have significant elevations in certain cytokines (chemicals that moderate immune and inflammatory responses). The cytokine increases, according to the researchers, accompanied and accounted for increases in abdominal discomfort, headache, and joint and muscle pain—symptoms that are obviously similar to those observed in CFS patients.

While a number of tests are purported to uncover food intolerances, there is no substitute for the elimination and challenge diet. The aim of the elimination and challenge diet is the removal of certain food and chemicals (reported as causing a sensitivity) for a period of at least ten days. Most often, this means the removal of wheat, corn, dairy, egg, gluten, tomato, caffeine, aspartame, monosodium glutamate, food dyes, and preservatives such as benzoates. During the challenge phase, the individual is placed on a "few-foods" diet, where hypoallergenic foods such as lamb, turkey, rice, pears, apples, sweet potatoes, and lentils are allowed and rotated (not taken on consecutive days). After at least ten days, the suspect foods are introduced into the diet one group at a time (three to four glasses of milk for three days, then yogurt, cheese, etc.), waiting at least three days before introducing a new group and looking for any significant change in symptoms. Keeping a diet diary during the challenge/reintroduction phase is an important tool and will be helpful for you and your nutritionally oriented medical doctor (MD) or licensed naturopathic physician (ND). An MD or ND should supervise an elimination and challenge diet because such a professional is best suited to interpret the signs and symptoms that may result.

Table 7. Wheat and dairy alternatives.

Wheat Alternatives: Amaranth	Kasha	Quinoa	Rye
Barley	Millet	Rice	Tapioca
Buckwheat	Oats		
Dairy Alternatives: Soy beverages/cheeses/yogurts			
Rice beverages/cheeses/yogurts			
Almond beverages			
Oat beverages			
Note: In considering a milk alternative, choose beverages fortified with calcium, vitamins A&D and vitamin B12.			

In conclusion, food intolerances and/or the intolerances to chemicals within foods and beverages may be playing a role in the symptoms of CFS and FM. Recent research has uncovered a physiological mechanism by which food intolerances can cause symptoms that resemble some of those that are observed in CFS. Given that many CFS and FM patients report new and increased sensitivity after illness onset, including food sensitivities, it may be worthwhile to attempt dietary modifications in an effort to manage symptoms. There are a number of unscientific devices and methods purported to uncover food intolerances; however, there is no substitute for an elimination and challenge diet, and this attempt should be conducted under the supervision of a nutritionally oriented doctor.

ADDITIONAL CONSIDERATIONS

In the past few years there have been a number of published reports in quality medical journals indicating that a vegetarian or vegan (no animal products) diet may alleviate some of the symptoms of FM. Specifically, adhering to such diets resulted in significant improvements in joint stiffness, pain, sleep, exercise tolerance, vitality, mental, and overall health. The positive effects of these diets have a sound scientific basis—according to research published in the *American Journal of Clinical Nutrition*, vegetarian diets increase antioxidant status in the blood, something critically important to those with CFS/FM. In addition, a vegetarian diet increases magnesium intake, an essential mineral found to be low in both CFS and FM, and can increase plasma glutathione, one of the body's most important detoxifying chemicals. In contrast to fruits and vegetables, a diet high in meat tends to promote inflammation and an acidic environment in the body.

With such impressive results in the published research, perhaps you might be thinking of becoming a vegetarian or vegan. It is important to point out that despite reductions in pain, improved vitality, and other positive outcomes, very few patients continued on the diets after the conclusion of the trials. Compliance with dietary modifications can be difficult and time-consuming, and can be a hindrance in social situations, draining energy that, in a CFS/FM patient, just isn't there in the first place. The research indicates that the benefits of the vegetarian diet in FM are more likely to be a result of the *inclusion* of plant-based nutrients rather than the elimination of meat. I suggest that CFS/FM patients can benefit from a *reduction* in meat intake and an increase in the consumption of fish as a healthy protein along with phytochemical-filled fruits and vegetables.

Finally, numerous Web sites promote the elimination of nightshade vegetables (eggplant, bell and hot peppers, tomato, and potato) in arthritis, mostly as a result of a small study published in 1993. However, despite the popular claims, there is no published research indicating that these foods are aggravating in FM, and don't forget that permanent removal eliminates intake of some healthy phytochemicals. That said, an elimination and challenge of nightshade foods in both CFS/FM might be worth a try, particularly with our research showing a small percentage (17 percent) of CFS patients reporting aggravation from tomatoes.

CHAPTER SUMMARY

- Despite the convenience, frozen dinners and fast food should be kept to an absolute minimum.
- CFS/FM patients should be eating vegetables in abundance and a minimum of two servings of fruits per day.
- Vegetables and fruits provide phytochemicals that perform numerous functions in the body, including acting as potent antioxidants and protecting the nervous system.
- Soft drinks, both with sugar and without, should be avoided in CFS/FM.
- Dietary omega-3 fatty acids are very important to CFS/FM patients. Excellent sources are fish, flax seeds, canola oil, and walnuts.

- Intolerances to food and the chemicals in them may play a role in CFS/FM symptoms. An elimination and challenge diet, supervised by a doctor, is the most appropriate way to identify potential food sensitivities.
- A reduction of meat and an increase in fish and legumes is encouraged.

CHAPTER FIVE

DIETARY SUPPLEMENTS AND HERBS

When I first started consulting with Dr. Bested's CFS/FM patients a number of years ago, it quickly became clear that many were self-prescribing a wide variety of "natural" products. Most of the products that patients were listing were being marketed heavily but had very little in the way of science to support their use in CFS/FM. Everywhere CFS/FM patients turn, there is a magic-bullet supplement that is purported to turn the illness around. Patients with chronic illnesses like CFS/FM are easy targets because they are so desperate to be well, so desperate to gain some semblance of their former lives. What's another $29.99 or even $89.99 for a cure? It seems like a small price to pay! Internet sites bombard CFS/FM patients with a host of different products.

We decided to research the types and amounts of dietary-herbal supplements that were being consumed by patients. Dr. Bested and I presented our findings to the scientific community at the Sixth International Conference on CFS, FM and Related Illnesses in February 2003 in Washington, D.C. More than 90 percent of patients from our metro Toronto sample reported consuming supplements on a *regular* basis—everything from multivitamins to elaborate detoxification protocols. The patients who reported regular consumption of dietary/herbal supplements had an average intake of six various supplements per day, with some taking as many as twenty-four different remedies per day. We were initially hoping to get some clues as to which, if any, might be helping with symptoms. However, with the exception of a multivitamin, fish oil, and evening primrose oil, there was little consistency among the types of supplement consumed. Incredibly, there were 109 *different* types of dietary supplements and herbal remedies consumed on a regular basis.

The bottom line is that the so-called "natural product industry" as it exists today in North America is much like the old "wild west," with little to no regulation. There are also massive gaps between the marketing of products and scientific data on their safety and effectiveness. Questions regarding quality assurance and truth in labelling are continually being raised. On numerous occasions it has been found that the ingredients that are claimed on a supplement bottle are not reflective of what is actually in the bottle. Thankfully, change is in the works. The Canadian government has recently introduced new regulations on natural products that will more strictly govern claims. It is likely that other countries, including the United States, will follow this lead.

Despite the shortcomings, I do appreciate that CFS/FM patients have accessibility to nutritional and herbal products that may have therapeutic value, and I do believe (and much more importantly, some science shows) that a number of these products can be very helpful. However, the supplements of real value are a minority in the vast "sea of supplements," and none of them are a cure.

Let's have a look at some of the supplements that may be valuable in general health and *management* of symptoms.

MULTIVITAMIN-MINERAL SUPPLEMENT

Although there is no research to indicate that taking a multivitamin-mineral, or "multi," will directly improve the symptoms of CFS/FM, all patients should be supplementing with a quality multi for general health purposes. Researchers from Harvard Medical School have reviewed the evidence surrounding the use of vitamins and published their findings in the *Journal of the American Medical Association* (2002). They concluded that taking a multi may offer protection against a variety of chronic illnesses and, in the accompanying editorial, went on to suggest that all adults should be taking a multi on a regular basis. It is understood that a multi is not a substitute for a well-balanced, nutritious diet—it is, however, a kind of "insurance policy" that all essential nutrients are taken in at adequate levels. Given the research showing that CFS/FM patients have decreased levels of a variety of nutrients, I feel it is even more important for patients to take a good-quality multi.

With such a wide variety of multivitamin-mineral formulas on the market, consumers are often understandably confused about what constitutes a quality product. Many CFS/FM patients are surprised to learn that some well-known multi brands contain commercial food dyes such as FD&C yellow #6, aluminum lake, sugars, gums, starches, and fillers. Based on the limited research available, which I reviewed in the nutrition chapter, CFS/FM patients should avoid artificial additives as much as possible. Another consideration when looking for a good multivitamin-mineral formula is finding one that contains adequate levels of nutrients and yet at the same time avoiding unnecessary and potentially toxic "mega-doses" of vitamins and minerals.

Additional supplementation with calcium and magnesium may be required because they are bulky minerals and most multi-vitamin-mineral formulas do not provide adequate levels. Some CFS experts suggest that physiological changes brought about by the illness may result in increased loss of calcium from the bones. In addition, CFS and FM patients often have a condition called small intestinal bacterial overgrowth (discussed in detail below) that can also interfere with bone mineralization. This, coupled with the post-illness decline in physical activity, suggests CFS/FM patients should be very diligent in ensuring they have adequate calcium intake. Certain nutrients that may be of value will be discussed separately.

OMEGA-3 FATTY ACIDS AND GAMMA-LINOLENIC ACID

If you have already read chapter 4, then you know how important omega-3 fatty acids are in human nutrition and health. The current ratio of dietary omega-6 to omega-3 is upwards of 15-20:1 when it should be closer to 1:1. Essential fatty acids in general, and omega-3 fatty acids in particular, have been the subject of intense scientific research. While the research has been conflicting, supplementation with essential fatty acids may be a means to reduce the symptoms of CFS/FM. Gamma-linolenic acid (GLA) is an omega-6 fatty acid derived from evening primrose oil, bor-

Table 1. National Academy of Sciences Institute of Medicine, adult dietary reference intakes (with known upper limits).

Folic acid	1000 mcg	Iodine	1100 mcg
Niacin	35 mg	Iron	45 mg
Vitamin B6	100 mg	Magnesium	350 mg
Vitamin A	3000 mcg	Manganese	11 mg
Vitamin C	2000 mg	Molybdenum	2000 mcg
Vitamin D	50 mcg	Nickel	1 mg
Vitamin E	1000 mg	Phosphorus	4000 mg
Choline	3500 mg	Selenium	400 mcg
Boron	20 mg	Vanadium	1.8 mg
Calcium	2500 mg	Zinc	40 mg
Copper	10 mg	Water	3.7 L male
Fluoride	10 mg		2.7 L female

age oil, and black currant oil, but it has some special properties that the other omega-6 predominant oils such as corn, sunflower, and safflower lack. In contrast to the other omega-6 oils, GLA has been shown to have potent anti-inflammatory properties and may be of value in a number of medical conditions, particularly in women's health and rheumatoid arthritis. Published research shows that a 4 g combination of fish oil and GLA (in a 4:1 ratio of fish to GLA) is helpful in improving the symptoms of CFS. After 3 months, 85 percent of the CFS patients had improved versus 17 percent of placebo controls. This important ratio of fish oil to GLA from primrose oil is commercially available in supplement form as Efamol. See the Appendix for details. In addition, a small study published in the *International Journal of Clinical Pharmacology and Therapeutics* (2000) indicates that 4.5 g of fish oil daily can improve pain, fatigue, and depression in FM patients.

As CFS/FM patients often experience depression related to having a chronic illness, it is important to note recent studies that show the value of essential fatty acids in the treatment of depression. There are two main omega-3 fatty acids in fish oil, namely docosahexanoic acid (DHA) and eicosapentanoic (EPA), and while both are essential in human health, it is the EPA component that seems to be of value as an anti-inflammatory agent and in alleviating depression. Placebo-controlled studies published in two prestigious journals, the *American Journal of Psychiatry* and *Archives of General Psychiatry* in 2002, indicate that adding fish oil (pure EPA) to conventional antidepressant medications can be of great value. The latter study used various doses and found that 1 g of EPA daily may be most therapeutic, even more so than higher doses. Pure DHA and mixed DHA/EPA supplements do not seem to be as effective in treating depression, and it has been suggested that a DHA/EPA mixture may interfere with the effectiveness of the EPA alone. Most fish oil products on the market are mixed DHA and EPA; however, pure EPA supplements are now available in North America—one such product is o3mega+ joy, which is available throughout Canada in supermarkets, pharmacies, and health food stores and elsewhere over the Internet. For more information, see the Appendix. One significant advantage of o3mega+ joy is that it is specially coated to open after it passes through the stomach. By not opening in the acidic environment of the stomach, the consumer avoids the upset stomach and "fishy repeat" that is so common with standard fish oil capsules. The research on EPA and its apparent ability to enhance the effectiveness of prescription drugs is an exciting development that requires follow-up. There is no question that omega-3 fatty acids play a critical role in proper functioning of the nervous system; however, it is critically important that omega-3 fatty acids not be considered a substitute for appropriate mental health care and medications.

The EPA omega-3 from fish oil appears to be a strong candidate for the treatment of CFS. A series of case reports published in the journal *Prostaglandins, Leukotrienes and Essential Fatty Acids* (2004) by United Kingdom essential fatty acid expert Dr. Basant Puri, indicate EPA can improve the symptoms of CFS. Amazingly, in one case report published in the *International*

Journal of Clinical Practice (2004), Dr. Puri shows that improvements in CFS symptoms with 930 mg of EPA, 290 mg DHA, and 100 mg GLA daily over sixteen weeks were associated with a reduction in the size of the free spaces in the brain (ventricles). Enlarged ventricles have been found among CFS patients and may indicate accelerated breakdown of important components within the brain cells called phospholipids. This suggests that EPA is having an effect in maintaining the normal brain structure in CFS. This patient had improvements in mood, mobility, and sleep.

Fish oil supplementation has an excellent record of safety and has been used in large trials, some spanning three years, with few reports of significant adverse effects. However, when taking a supplement or over-the-counter remedy, you should discuss it with your health care provider. Fish oil may have a mild blood-thinning effect, and while initial research showed that borage oil may increase blood platelet aggregation (thicken blood and prevent efficient circulation), more recent research shows that doses up to 3000 mg a day have no effect on platelets.

PROBIOTICS

The term "probiotic therapy" generally refers to the use of viable bacteria to positively influence the health of the gastrointestinal tract. I will outline a number of reasons why probiotic therapy may be of particular value in CFS/FM. First, though, a little background on the "State of the Intestines" in CFS/FM as we know it.

The overlap between CFS/FM and irritable bowel syndrome is well-documented, and most patients with both CFS and FM report significant gastrointestinal (GI) complaints after onset of the illness. Irritable bowel syndrome is characterized by abdominal pain, discomfort, bloating, distension, and diarrhea or constipation or both. CFS/FM patients describe many of these symptoms, and research indicates that all is not normal inside the GI tracts of those with these conditions. Indeed, research shows that the majority of patients with CFS, FM, and the often-related women's health condition endometriosis have a condition called small intestinal bacterial overgrowth (SIBO). In addition, both CFS/FM and irritable bowel syndrome are conditions that may involve a reduction in the numbers of anaerobic bacteria, including beneficial lactobacilli and bifidobacteria.

There are more living bacteria in the gastrointestinal tract than there are cells in the human body, but the majority of these bacteria are present in the large intestine or colon. When a migration of bacteria from the large intestine into the small intestine occurs, or when bacteria do not "move on down the line," so to speak, the condition of SIBO can wreak havoc on GI function. Bacterial overgrowth in the small intestine can cause many of the previously described GI symptoms, and when present in excess in the small intestine, bacteria can produce toxic substances and interfere with the absorption of important nutrients. Despite a diet that is pretty much the same as the standard American diet (catch that acronym? *SAD!*), CFS patients have been shown to have lower levels of B vitamins and other important nutrients. Patients with both irritable bowel syndrome and CFS have been shown to have abnormalities in the proper passage of food along the GI tract (motility disturbances) that may be a cause for the development of SIBO. Dr. Mark Pimentel and his colleagues from Cedars-Sinai Medical Center in Los Angeles have had great short-term success treating IBS, CFS, and FM patients with SIBO using antibiotics.

There is a relatively simple test to assess for SIBO, the lactulose hydrogen breath test. When lactulose is consumed, it is not absorbed; intestinal bacteria ferment it, and hydrogen gas is produced. A doctor can review your test results and determine if you have an early rise in hydrogen, indicating potential bacterial overgrowth in the small intestine. See www.thedoctors.ca for more information on the lactulose hydrogen breath test.

If SIBO is determined, it will be necessary to take antibiotics for effective treatment. The co-administration of probiotics along with prescription antibiotics when treating SIBO is necessary because:

1. Antibiotics can have significant and long-term effects on the normal GI bacterial flora (i.e., the good lactobacilli and bifidobacteria).

2. Research published in the *American Journal of Gastro-enterology* and the *European Journal of Gastroenterology and Hepatology* shows that prior antibiotic use is associated with the onset of irritable bowel syndrome and subsequent bowel symptoms of unknown origin.

3. Research presented by Australian researchers Henry Butt and colleagues shows that CFS and FM patients already have diminished numbers of healthy anaerobic bacteria such as bifidobacteria in the colon. Antibiotics may worsen this situation.

4. Various strains of lactobacillus and bifidobacterium have themselves been shown to treat SIBO and suppress even difficult-to-treat organisms such as ulcer-causing *Helicobacter pylori*. Probiotics can produce lactic acid and other directly antimicrobial compounds in the bowel. Controlled studies have also found various strains of probiotics to be helpful in the treatment of irritable bowel syndrome, a condition where SIBO is prevalent.

5. When probiotics are co-administered along with multiple antibiotics in the treatment of ulcer-causing *Helicobacter pylori*, patients report a lower incidence of side effects such as diarrhea, nausea, and taste disturbance. This is important because, once started, antibiotics should be finished, and any agents that can increase compliance will reduce antibiotic resistance, an alarming global trend.

6. Probiotics may prevent a recurrence of SIBO by regulating bowel movements.

The research by Dr. Henry Butt and his colleagues is groundbreaking because they were able to make a connection between low levels of anaerobic bacteria and high levels of aerobic bacteria (particularly enterococci) with the cognitive difficulties of

CFS and FM. It remains to be seen if this is cause or effect in CFS/FM or if normalizing the intestinal flora (bacteria) in CFS/FM will have any significant effect on the gastrointestinal and cognitive symptoms of the illnesses. Interestingly, when Dr. Pimentel and his team eradicated the bacterial overgrowth in the small intestines of CFS patients, they noticed improvements in memory, concentration, pain, and depression. Intestinal bacteria, both good and bad, is an exciting and emerging area of research. It is clear that these tiny microbes can have significant effects beyond the gastrointestinal tract. A recent study published in the *American Journal of Clinical Nutrition* showed that a lactobacillus strain given orally could reduce the presence of undesirable bacteria in the nasal passages of adults. Separate research has shown that oral probiotics can beneficially alter vaginal microflora and lower levels of the yeast *Candida albicans*. The particular strains that can do this are L. rhamnosus GR-1 and L. fermentum, highly researched at the University of Western Ontario and soon to be on the North American market.

It is also clear from both animal and human research that stress can have a detrimental effect on the beneficial intestinal bacteria, particularly lactobacilli and bifidobacteria. In contrast, the administration of a probiotic-multivitamin compound to adults with stress or exhaustion has been shown to lead to significant reductions in stress, frequency of infections, and gastrointestinal discomfort over the six-month study (published in *Advances in Therapy*, 2002). A symbiotic relationship appears to exist between probiotics and omega-3 fatty acids. In separate animal studies, polyunsaturated fatty acid supplementation (fish oil in particular) enhances the growth of intestinal lactobacilli and bifidobacteria, and in turn, the administration of probiotics can enhance cellular omega-3 fatty acid levels.

Hopefully, further research will determine if the administration of probiotics is specifically of benefit to CFS/FM. In the meantime, given the research documenting altered intestinal bacteria in these illnesses and the large volumes of international research supporting lactobacilli and bifidobacteria in human health, probiotics should be considered a worthwhile supplement. Here are some of the documented benefits of lactobacilli and bifidobacteria:

- Vitamin synthesis
- Stimulation of cellular immunity
- Protection of the intestinal barrier, ensuring only appropriate nutrients pass through the intestines to the blood
- Production of short chain fatty acids, fuel for intestinal cells
- Break down potentially cancer-causing substances
- Lower the levels of potentially neurotoxic (nerve-damaging) compounds
- Act as potent antioxidants
- Increase levels of omega-3 fatty acids in cell membranes
- Increase natural killer cell activity
- May diminish allergies

Probiotics have an exceptional record of safety, and despite the huge increase in commercial preparations, there has been no rise in negative reports due to lactobacilli and bifidobacteria. One of the main problems with probiotics is finding a brand that has therapeutic levels of viable bacteria inside the bottle. There are a number of reports in the United States and Canada where independent testing revealed very few live bacteria in store-purchased formulas and commercial yogurt.

Another problem is the marketing of preparations (that may or may not have live bacteria) under the umbrella term acidophilus—and using the research of other strains to promote the product. There are three main features to a probiotic name: genus, species, and strain. For example, Lactobacillus (genus) casei (species) Shirota (strain) or Lactobacillus rhamnosus GR-1 are well-documented bacteria with at least partially known physiological and biological activities. Consumers need to look for probiotic formulas that have identified strains of bacteria, strains that have been the subject of scientific and medical research.

Is there a CFS/FM probiotic of choice?

For now there is no specific strain that has been shown to help CFS/FM. However, among the strains that may be of value in CFS/FM include Lactobacillus GG (Con Agra), which is marketed as Culturelle™ in North America, and Yakult *Lactobacillus casei Shirota* (LcS). *Lactobacillus GG* is an excellent probiotic which has been shown in clinical research to limit allergies. Yakult LcS may emerge as the ideal probiotic for CFS/FM. When my colleagues and I published the rationale for the use of probiotics in CFS/FM (*Medical Hypotheses*, 2003) there was one strain that immediately came to mind and it was LcS. The reason is that LcS has extensive research in regulating bowel function and has been shown clinically to improve immune status, including natural killer cell activity. In addition, because of its effects on immune chemicals called cytokines, LcS may have far-reaching effects beyond the gut and ultimately influence inflammation, mood, and essential fatty acid status. LcS is worth a try. It is hoped that LcS will become widely available in the future; for now it is available as a fermented skim milk drink at select Japanese grocery stores in California and New York. The drink is simply known as Yakult (pronounced *yakoultoe*) and each small bottle of the probiotic beverage contains 8 billion colony-forming units of live LcS. You can contact Yakult USA (see the Appendix) for availability and a store that may be willing to ship product.

The Web site www.usprobiotics.org maintains an up-to-date catalog of researched strains that have documented health benefits.

ANTIOXIDANTS

The fact that CFS/FM patients are under increased oxidative stress and have a diminished antioxidant capacity has been discussed elsewhere in this book. The research in this area keeps piling up and suggests that supplementation with antioxidant formulas is therapeutically valuable. There is some preliminary research indicating that antioxidants may be something to consider.

Two small, double-blind, placebo-controlled studies suggest that antioxidants may be of value in CFS/FM. One paper appeared in the *Journal of Nutritional and Environmental Medicine* and showed that 80 mg of anthocyanidin (a polyphenol-phyto-chemical derived from grape seed, cranberry, and bilberry) daily could improve sleep quality and fatigue in FM. In a separate study involving a Swedish pollen extract (Polbax) high in antioxidant polyphenols, administration of the product to twenty-two patients for three months resulted in significant improvements in the treatment group vs. placebo. Improvements were noted in fatigue, sleep disturbance, GI complaints, and hypersensitivity. There were some objective physiological signs that the antioxidant formula was working; the extract resulted in a more stable red blood cell count with diminished signs of oxidative stress.

In addition, one preliminary trial involving CFS patients used intramuscular injections of one of the body's most potent antioxidants—glutathione. The results of the six-month trial were remarkable, with 82 percent reporting improvements in fatigue and 71 percent reporting improvements in memory and concentration. Our colleague, board-certified neurologist Dr. David Perlmutter of Naples, Florida, is an expert in the use of intravenous (IV) glutathione for CFS and other medical conditions involving the CNS. For further information on the use of glutathione in neurological conditions, including an instructional video for your physician to administer IV glutathione appropriately, see Dr. Perlmutter's Web site at www.brainrecovery.com. Indications are that IV glutathione may be even more effective than the intra-muscular delivery.

A recent open-label study (i.e., no placebo group) showed that 200 mg of Co-enzyme Q10 and 200 mg of ginkgo biloba daily for three months might be of benefit. The study involved twenty-three patients with FM, and the results showed that the combination improved quality of life scores, and 64 percent of patients reported overall improvement at the conclusion of the study. Both Co-Q10 and ginkgo are well-documented potent antioxidants, particularly in the nervous system; in addition, Co-

Q10 can boost cellular energy, and ginkgo can improve circulation to the brain.

Our friends from the Panjab University Institute of Pharmaceutical Sciences in India have shown that, in the animal model of CFS, the administration of various antioxidants can significantly reduce oxidative stress and increase glutathione levels. These researchers showed that the administration of antioxidants was also effective in increasing the antioxidant status within the brains of the animals. The antioxidants used in the study included the drug carvedilol, the Indian herb ashwagandha (Withania somnifera), quercetin, melatonin (discussed below), and St. John's wort (Hypericum perforatum, discussed below). Ashwagandha has a 2,500-year history as a central nervous system tonic and an adaptogen (herb that helps one adapt to stress) in India, and St. John's wort is well-known as a mood-regulating herb. Many people are surprised to learn that these herbs and melatonin are powerful antioxidants. Ashwagandha may be of particular value in CFS/FM. Many animal studies have shown that it has anti-stress activities in both acute and chronic models of experimental stress. In addition, ashwagandha enhances cognitive activity in Alzheimer's disease models, has anti-anxiety and antidepressive activities, and promotes antioxidant activities in the brains of animals. Although ashwagandha has a long history of safe use in the Indian sub-continent, human trials are lacking; hopefully clinical trials will determine if ashwagandha is effective for patients with CFS/FM.

The small trials involving antioxidants are encouraging and certainly require follow-up; it is critical that companies involved in the sales of such products make an effort to invest in this area of research. As you know, it costs a ton of money to be on TV for a half an hour hawking some product—coral calcium, CFS/FM cures with pine bark, or whatever. I challenge these companies to invest some of these dollars into university-based research where the results will be published regardless of the outcome. One Canadian company, Ehn Inc., has an established track record of supporting university-based research on products they bring to market. Most notably, greens+, a multiple-ingredient, powdered "green" food supplement has been shown in two separate University of Toronto human studies to boost antioxidant levels and increase energy and vitality in otherwise healthy adults. For more, please see the sidebar.

In any case, patients are suffering in the here and now, and antioxidants may help in symptom reduction. Clinical experience shows that the administration of antioxidants to CFS/FM patients can produce some improvement. Our recommendations

---

The Research on Greens+

Greens+ was formulated by nutrition expert Sam Graci about ten years ago. Since then it has become a bestseller in Canada, with numerous testimonials over the years claiming that it increases energy and vitality. I am a skeptic when it comes to testimonials, and so are university-based scientists. Therefore, researchers at the University of Toronto asked the distributor of greens+ to put the product to the test. The subjects, one hundred otherwise healthy women from Toronto, were instructed to take either greens+ or a carefully matched placebo powdered beverage for three months. Subjects were evaluated using various validated questionnaires.

After the three months, those taking the greens+ did indeed have increased energy over the placebo group. The results are very encouraging. In separate published research, greens+ increased blood antioxidant levels and lowered oxidative stress in otherwise healthy adults from Toronto. According to the University of Toronto researchers, the beneficial phytonutrients (polyphenols) in greens+ are well-absorbed. This is useful information because studies have not always shown that supplemental polyphenols are well-absorbed. An additional potential benefit for CFS/FM patients is that greens+ has been shown in University of Toronto research to stimulate osteoblasts, the cells that are critical in bone formation and maintenance. While the clinical work involved healthy adults, the encouraging results indicate potential benefit in CFS/FM.

for potentially therapeutic supplemental antioxidants are listed below. Keep in mind, though, that the word *supplement* should be taken literally: they are a supplement to a healthy diet—the intake of *dietary* antioxidants should be prioritized. The research on the effects of antioxidant-containing foods (as discussed in chapter 4) indicates they are much more robust than supplements.

Antioxidants work in synergy, much like an orchestra, so when supplementing, it is important to take a formula that has multiple antioxidants. The vast array of phytochemicals and antioxidants that exist in nature has different and complementary mechanisms of action in the body. Research is beginning to show the benefits of taking antioxidants together. For example, isoflavones from soy and other plants have increased antioxidant activity in the presence of vitamin C, and the antioxidant activity of both alfalfa extract and isoflavones have dramatically increased antioxidant activity in the presence of Acerola cherry extract. Many researchers are beginning to look at how whole food extracts and herbal extracts work together.

There is no evidence that consuming large amounts (up to ten servings per day) of fruits and vegetables is unsafe. There is, however, test-tube research indicating that *isolated* antioxidants, such as vitamin C, can act as pro-oxidants (i.e., increase your oxidative stress) under certain laboratory conditions. Isolated antioxidants can have what are referred to as bi-phasic properties, meaning that at a certain level they can have strong antioxidant properties, but at another they may actually *increase* oxidative stress.

One reason why there seems to be no evidence against whole foods may again be due to synergy of plant-based phytochemicals. Recent research published in the *Journal of Pharmacy and Pharmacology* showed that when antioxidants are taken together, the pro-oxidant effects (in this case of vitamin C) are negated by the presence of the other antioxidants. The same research also showed that two antioxidants together have greater antioxidant potential than the sum of the two individually. It appears that there is not only an increase in effectiveness but also safety through combining antioxidant therapy.

If you choose to supplement with an antioxidant formula, here are our recommendations based on research and experience:

1. Inform your doctor.
2. Start with low doses.
3. Keep the synergistic activity of antioxidants in mind and choose a formula(s) with a broad range of antioxidant nutrients and plant-based (phyto) chemicals.
4. Beyond the traditional vitamins A, C, and E, some of the antioxidant ingredients that may be of benefit include coenzyme Q10, bilberry, ginkgo biloba, ashwagandha, oligomeric proanthocyanidins from grape seeds, alpha-lipoic acid, N-acetylcysteine, acetyl-L-carnitine, selenium, soy isoflavones, the flavonoids in cocoa powder, and the catechins of green tea. These antioxidants may not only protect the blood vessels and nerve cells from oxidative damage, they also have the ability to protect and improve the function of the "energy packets of the cell," the mitochondria. Coenzyme Q10 and acetyl-L-carnitine may be particularly effective in CFS/FM for this purpose. Although L-glutathione is the most promising of the antioxidants, oral administration is ineffective. As mentioned, administration of intra-muscular or intravenous glutathione may be helpful for some patients.
5. Cysteine is an amino acid that is essential for the maintenance of the body's own glutathione supply. Consider a quality, cysteine-rich, whey protein supplement not only as a good, usually well-tolerated protein to add to the diet but also to help boost and maintain glutathione levels. Research published in the *European Journal of Clinical Investigation* and the *European Journal of Nutrition* indicates that there is little difference between expensive multilevel-market whey protein and a quality whey protein (manufac-

tured by standard procedures) in their ability to boost blood glutathione levels. Proteins+ is a high-quality, cysteine-rich whey product currently manufactured in Canada.

NICOTINAMIDE ADENINE DINUCLEOTIDE (NADH)

Widely available in North America, NADH is a natural co-enzyme that is specially prepared so that it maintains oral stability. It is reported to improve the production of cellular energy by boosting the levels of adenine triphosphate (ATP). It is well known that ATP is the fuel source for cellular energy, and there is no question NADH that occurs naturally in the human body is crucial in the production of energy. It seems reasonable, then, that NADH supplementation may be of value in conditions such as CFS where cellular energy is less than optimal. Indeed, ENADA® has been the subject of a small but well-designed clinical trial involving CFS patients at Georgetown University. This pilot study, using 10 mg daily, showed that 31 percent of the CFS patients had improvement in various symptoms versus 8 percent of the placebo group.

As a result of the pilot study, numerous Web sites sprung up selling and promoting NADH as the magic bullet for CFS (and a host of other neuropsychiatric illnesses). This typical "coral-calcium-esque" marketing continues. Clinical experience indicates that NADH may be most useful when *combined* with other antioxidants. Remember that antioxidants interact with each other, working in a synergistic fashion. Bottom line, NADH is a potent antioxidant and may offer some benefit when combined with other plant- and nutrient-based antioxidants in CFS/FM symptom reduction.

MAGNESIUM AND MALIC ACID

There have been some reports in the medical literature suggesting that magnesium may be of value in the treatment of CFS and FM. Magnesium is involved in more than three hundred enzyme reactions in the human body and is essential in energy production. Magnesium is of particular importance to the health of the central nervous system, as low levels of magnesium (and high levels of aluminum) are associated with dementia. Research published in the journal *Lancet* showed that CFS patients had low levels of magnesium and that intra-muscular injections with magnesium were helpful in treatment. Other researchers have published findings in the *Journal of the American Dietetic Association* (1996) and the *International Journal of Neuroscience* (2003) indicating that more CFS patients have low levels of red blood cells and serum magnesium than controls. Belgian researchers suggest that some CFS patients have "subclinical" magnesium deficiency—there are no overt symptoms of magnesium deficiency and lab values may be within normal range, yet magnesium intake, absorption, and bioavailability may be clinically relevant to a variety of symptoms.

In the case of FM, the investigations into magnesium levels have also drawn inconsistent results. The long and the short of it is that there appears to be some abnormalities in magnesium metabolism. A placebo-controlled study published in the *Journal of Rheumatology* using magnesium (450 mg) and malic acid (1,200 mg) did not show any clear value in reducing the symptoms of FM. Malic acid is a fruit acid that is found in high amounts in apples; its chemical anion form malate is critical in cellular energy production. Interestingly, when the placebo arm of the study was discontinued and participants were put on labelled doses up to 900 mg of magnesium and 2,400 mg of malic acid, there were significant improvements in FM symptoms. Placebo effect? Probably, but only further research will determine if the dose in the controlled study was too low. In the clinical setting, many patients report that the magnesium/malic acid combination is a helpful one. Perhaps magnesium and/or malic acid may be most helpful to a subset of CFS and FM patients.

In the meantime, we do know that oral magnesium has been shown to be effective in the management of migraine headaches and a number of symptoms associated with premenstrual syndrome—both of which are common coexisting conditions in CFS/FM. Low levels of magnesium intake are associated with osteoporosis, heart disease, and diabetes. Given that magnesium intake is generally lower than recommended in Western countries and is important in so many aspects of human health, I recommend ensuring a supplementary intake of 350 mg per day for adolescents and adults. This is the supplement dose (separate from dietary intake through food and water) set by the National Academy of Sciences as the tolerable upper limit (UL). The UL is defined as the level that is likely to pose no risk of adverse effects. Taking higher doses may be of value in CFS/FM but requires the supervision of a nutritionally oriented medical or naturopathic physician. Don't expect your magnesium intake to be covered by your multivitamin-mineral formula—most multi formulas on the market have only minimal levels of calcium and magnesium because they are bulky minerals.

CALCIUM

Due to physiological changes brought on by the illness and decreased physical activities as a result of the illness, CFS/FM patients need to take extra care to ensure adequate calcium intake. Research indicates that FM is indeed a risk factor for osteoporosis in adulthood; patients have been shown to have decreased bone mineral density, particularly in the spine. At the time of this writing, there have been no investigations into the bone mineral density of CFS patients, although a recent article in *Medical Hypotheses* provided a sound rationale as to why the physiological changes induced by the illness would negatively affect bone density. CFS patients may have increased demands for calcium at the expense of bone storage and increased bone break down along with decreased bone formation for the following reasons:

1. Deregulation of the RNase L antiviral pathway and associated abnormalities of the tiny channels in cells through which calcium flows.

2. The presence of the organism *Mycoplasma fermentans*, which produces something called MALP-2, which can increase bone break down.

3. Lower levels of insulin-like growth factor 1 (IGF-1) have been observed in some CFS patients. IGF-1 is essential in the production of bone-building cells called osteoblasts.

Calcium is deposited in the bone, as is money in a bank. The calcium levels in the blood are highly regulated to maintain acid/base balance. There is some research indicating that our modern diet, deficient in alkaline fruits and vegetables and top-heavy in acidic meats and grains, may be causing calcium to be leached out of the bone to maintain an appropriate pH in the blood. In addition to its importance in bone health, supplemental calcium has been shown to be of benefit in regulating blood pressure, lowering the risk of colon cancer, and reducing the symptoms of premenstrual syndrome. As with magnesium, there is no evidence that consuming calcium will have any tremendous effect on the symptoms of CFS/FM. However, given the importance of calcium in bone health and the illness-associated increased risk of osteoporosis in CFS/FM (direct physiology and lack of weight-bearing exercise), all CFS/FM patients should consider calcium supplementation. Adults should ensure an intake of at least 1,000 mg and those over fifty require at least 1,200 mg. The tolerable upper limit for calcium is 2,500 mg for adults, and unlike magnesium this level is based on diet *and* supplement intake combined.

FOLIC ACID AND VITAMINS B12 AND B6

Adequate levels of folic acid and vitamins B6 and B12 can be found in most quality multivitamin formulas, but a separate discussion on these two important B vitamins is worthwhile. Folic acid, vitamin B12, and vitamin B6 can all lower abnormally elevated levels of homocysteine. Elevated homocysteine is a well-known risk factor for heart disease and is correlated with poor cognitive performance. Researchers have found elevated levels of homocysteine in both CFS and FM. It is also interesting to note that a growing number of studies have linked elevated homocysteine and low levels of folic acid and vitamin B12 with clinical depression. In fact, a study in the *Journal of Affective Disorders* (2000) showed that just 500 mcg of folic acid added to the antidepressant Prozac could lead to a pronounced improvement in mood vs. placebo added to Prozac. Another recent study showed that higher levels of blood folic acid (folate) predicted a better outcome in depressed patients using antidepressant medications. The same has also been shown for B12; higher levels of B12 in the blood are associated with better recovery from depression.

It is understood that CFS/FM are separate and distinct from major depression. However, the findings of elevated homocysteine and the all-too-common illness-associated depressive symptoms are enough to suggest a trial of B vitamins in CFS/FM. It is important to note that both folic acid and B12 have been shown to lower homocysteine even when blood folate and B12 were considered "normal." The point is that just because "normal" levels of a nutrient are found in the blood, we cannot automatically assume that taking a supplement would be of no clinical value.

If you are fortunate enough to have a nutritionally oriented physician or naturopathic doctor licensed to perform intramuscular injections, then please give B12 and folic acid a try on a regular basis. I say this because absorption may be an issue in CFS/FM, and it is possible that intra-muscular injections are more effective than the oral route. If you do not have access to a doctor who will provide the injections, then at minimum, ensure you are taking in at least 400 mcg of supplemental folic acid and 500 mcg B12 daily along with 10 mg of vitamin B6. Note that B6 is a vitamin that not only assists folic acid and B12 in lowering homocysteine but also is essential in the normal production of brain neurotransmitters. Although I am recommending supplementary folic acid, B12, and B6, they are not a substitute for maximizing dietary intake. Any potential absorption issues that may be a factor should only encourage you to make every effort to eat a healthy diet. You know already that I am a fan of making dietary choices a priority over supplements, so I want to point out that a recent study in the *British Journal of Nutrition* (2003) showed a diet high in fresh berries, citrus fruits, and vegetables was able to increase blood folate levels and decrease homocysteine levels. Once again, food as medicine. Choosing deeply colored fruits and vegetables, whole grains, nuts, fish, and seafood ensures adequate intake of folic acid and vitamins B6 and B12. While much is made of red meat as the primary source of B12, salmon and seafood such as crabs, mussels, and clams contain more B12 per serving than cooked beef.

MELATONIN

Just as the moon and the oceans are in constant rhythm, so too is the human body. The circadian rhythms involve waxing and waning of core body temperature and spontaneous muscle (motor) activity. Melatonin is a hormone secreted by the brain's pineal gland in a twenty-four-hour circadian rhythm, regulating the sleep-wake cycle. Melatonin secretion normally increases about two hours before bedtime, peaks in the middle of the night, and drops thereafter. The rise and fall of melatonin is critical to the quality of human sleep. Research has shown that melatonin administration can enhance sleep when taken six hours before the natural peak—say 10:00 p.m. if the natural peak is 4:00 a.m. If the same dose of melatonin is taken in the morning, it can cause dizziness, drowsiness, and diminished daytime alertness. Research has focused mostly on insomnia due to shift work or jet lag. Interestingly, recent research has shown that melatonin is a potent antioxidant and has synergistic activity when co-administered with vitamins C and E.

What about CFS and FM; is there any potential value? The circadian rhythms have been shown to be disturbed in both CFS and FM. In fact, FM patients have been shown to have a 31 percent reduction in melatonin secretion at night versus healthy controls. In addition, the supplementation of 3 mg of melatonin to FM patients led to reduced tender point count, reduced pain, and improved sleep. Placebo effect cannot be ruled out, as this was an open-label trial where the patients knew they were taking melatonin. Despite these encouraging initial results and the finding of disturbed circadian rhythms in CFS, a controlled study involving CFS patients supplemented with 5 mg of melatonin for twelve weeks showed no difference over placebo. The study, published in the *European Journal of Clinical Investigation*, also showed that the light therapy known to help patients with seasonal affective disorder was of no value to CFS patients in reducing symptoms. Hopefully, future clinical research will examine melatonin supplementation along with antioxidants to determine if the combination may help to reduce symptoms.

As attractive as melatonin supplementation may seem, CFS/FM sleep disturbances are much more complex than jet lag and insomnia related to shift work. Much more research is required before melatonin can be routinely prescribed in CFS/FM. Even if there was convincing research that melatonin was of value in CFS/FM, I would not recommend self-prescription. There are some "natural" products that should be taken only under the supervision of a health care provider—I feel strongly that melatonin is one of them. Melatonin is certainly natural—it is a hormone—but that doesn't mean it's safe for regular consumption. Hormones work much like an orchestra; individual hormones can have a tremendous effect on the manufacture and secretion of other hormones. If you are considering giving melatonin a try, please see your MD, DO, or licensed ND for appropriate supervision.

S-ADENOSYL METHIONINE

Among the more than two hundred supplements that are marketed to CFS/FM patients, S-adenosyl methionine (SAMe) is actually the supplement with the highest level of evidence to support its use. A number of controlled trials have shown that both oral and intravenous SAMe is of value in the treatment of

FM. SAMe also has evidence to support its use in depression and rheumatoid and osteoarthritis, and may promote restful sleep. SAMe has been shown to support liver detoxification and improve antioxidant status by its ability to increase glutathione levels. Animal research has shown that SAMe can increase serotonin levels throughout the brain and may keep the nerve cells more "fluid" or flexible for proper neurotransmission.

SAMe may be a worthwhile supplement for CFS/FM patients; side effects are rare and usually consist of gastrointestinal disturbances, dry mouth, and restlessness. SAMe may have a mild blood-thinning effect. CFS/FM patients who are taking antidepressant medications or natural products such as 5-hydroxytryptophan, L-tryptophan, or Hypericum (St. John's wort) should only take SAMe under direct supervision of an MD, DO, or licensed ND. Keep in mind that therapeutic doses of SAMe are not cheap; when taking the 600 to 800 mg daily, as used in the FM trials, you can anticipate a bill of about seventy to a hundred dollars (U.S.) a month.

5-HYDROXYTRYPTOPHAN

Serotonin, the so-called "feel-good" brain chemical, is manufactured from the amino acid L-tryptophan. In simplistic terms, modern antidepressant drugs work by keeping more serotonin around for use at the nerve cells—they can prevent the breakdown of serotonin and prevent it from being placed back in storage. It would seem reasonable then that supplementing with the amino acid L-tryptophan may have a beneficial effect on mood by increasing serotonin levels. Indeed, a limited number of studies have shown that L-tryptophan may be helpful in treating depressive symptoms, anxiety, and insomnia and generally leads to a calming, mild sedation. Encouraging research, except there were big problems with L-tryptophan or, more specifically, a contaminated batch from Japan that was likely responsible for serious illness in more than fifteen hundred people and an estimated thirty deaths. The illness, eosinophilia myalgia syndrome (EMS), resulted in an FDA-issued recall in 1989, and L-tryptophan disappeared from the U.S. market—apparently never to return. L-tryptophan is available, and has been used safely, as a prescription item in Canada.

While the sun set on L-tryptophan in the United States, another related supplement (one step closer to serotonin) became a suitable replacement—5-hydroxytryptophan or 5-HTP for short. L-tryptophan gets converted into 5-HTP, which in turn gets converted into serotonin. 5-HTP has the advantage of readily passing through the highly regulated "security fence" around the brain called the blood-brain barrier (BBB). Only about 10 to 15 percent of L-tryptophan makes it through the barrier, and in the end, it is estimated that only 1 percent of dietary or supplemental L-tryptophan is converted into serotonin. In contrast, once through the BBB, 5-HTP is taken up by the nerve cells and completely converted into serotonin. As a result, the clinically effective doses of 5-HTP are much lower than those of L-tryptophan (around 200 mg versus 2 to 6 g of L-tryptophan).

There have been three clinical trials that have evaluated the use of 5-HTP in FM. Investigating 5-HTP in FM is certainly reasonable given that FM patients have been shown to have low levels of the L-tryptophan and serotonin activity. Two of the trials were higher quality, double-blind, placebo-controlled studies using either 300 mg or 400 mg of 5-HTP per day. Both of these studies showed that 5-HTP could reduce pain. In the study using 300 mg per day, there were also statistically significant reductions in morning stiffness, anxiety, and fatigue, as well as improved sleep. A third open-label study using 300 mg of 5-HTP found similar results when administered over ninety days.

5-HTP appears to be useful in a number of medical conditions. Other research has shown that it is beneficial in cases of depression, anxiety, insomnia, and migraine headaches. Despite the benefits, there are some words of caution regarding 5-HTP. Unless supervised by a doctor, it should not be taken with antidepressants because "serotonin syndrome," or overload of serotonin, may result. The symptoms of serotonin syndrome are euphoria, drowsiness, sustained rapid eye movement, overreaction of the reflexes, rapid muscle contraction and relaxation in the ankle causing abnormal movements of the foot, clumsiness, restlessness, feeling drunk and dizzy, muscle contraction and relaxation in the jaw, sweating, intoxication, muscle twitching, rigidity, and high body temperature. The typical side effects of 5-HTP taken within standard dosages are generally minimal and most often involve digestive upset. 5-HTP has not been associated with any outbreaks of illness due to contaminants, although one isolated case of EMS has been reported to be due to 5-HTP. A unique contaminant (Peak X) in 5-HTP is thought by some to be to blame for causing EMS in an adult and two children in one household. Two separate studies published in the *Journal of the American College of Nutrition* (2000) did not detect any Peak X or related impurities at all in commercial preparations of 5-HTP. In one of the studies, performed by researchers at Georgetown University, even the highest doses (ten times higher than typical human doses) were unable to cause EMS in animals. The second study concludes that there is no basis to doubt the safety of 5-HTP when it is derived from its natural source, *Griffonia* seed. Still, patients should contact the manufacturer to determine if they routinely assay for Peak X.

Instead of supplementing with 5-HTP, CFS/FM patients may want to consider taking in natural food-based tryptophan in the form of ZenBev™. This multipatented product includes pumpkinseed flour mixed with carbohydrate in the precise ratio required to get the tryptophan into the brain for conversion to serotonin. Although naturally high in tryptophan, pumpkin seeds alone will generally not be effective in boosting brain serotonin levels. Tryptophan will remain in the blood and not gain access through the blood-brain barrier and into the brain unless a specific ratio of carbohydrate is also consumed. After years of painstaking research, Toronto psychiatrist Craig Hudson and his team determined the proprietary blend of pumpkinseed flour and carbohydrate necessary to increase serotonin and melatonin for sleep. Early clinical trials using ZenBev™ are favorable in the areas of decreased anxiety and improved sleep. The powdered product may be an effective means to reduce symptoms, particularly in FM. See the Appendix for availability.

RHODIOLA ROSEA

This is probably the most exciting botanical to come to the North American market in recent years. Unlike many herbs, the clinical potential of rhodiola is backed up by some well-designed human studies. Rhodiola is an herb that has been studied intensively in Russian scientific laboratories over the last forty years. It has been used traditionally to enhance work performance and energy and decrease irritability under stressful conditions as well as physical and mental strain and viral exposure. Rhodiola is a classic adaptogen, and based on its historical use, particularly postviral/stress, it may be the most appropriate herb for CFS/FM patients. Rhodiola has been the subject of clinical research, the results of which seem to verify its traditional use.

Two double-blind, placebo-controlled trials of rhodiola extract appeared in Western scientific journals in 2000. The first study showed that the rhodiola group (170 mg per day) had statistically significant improvements in mental performance and measures of fatigue versus a placebo among medical doctors working night call rotations. The second trial involved medical students during a stressful exam period. The three-week study showed that those who received 100 mg of rhodiola had significant improvements in physical fitness, mental performance, sleep patterns, motivation to study, and general well-being. Those taking rhodiola also reported less need for sleep, greater mood stability, and reductions in mental fatigue versus those on placebo.

In 2003, a joint Russian-Swedish study showed that just one dose of rhodiola given during stressful conditions could improve mental function versus placebo. This study, again double-blind and placebo-controlled, showed that single doses of rhodiola

(370 mg or 555 mg) given at four o'clock in the morning could improve capacity for mental work and that rhodiola produces a pronounced antifatigue effect as reflected in an anti-fatigue index (AFI). While both doses were much more effective than placebo and a separate control group given no supplement at all, there was no significant difference in effect between the two doses. In fact there was a trend for the lower dose to be more effective. It seems that higher doses do not enhance the adaptogenic effects of rhodiola.

There have been no significant side effects noted for rhodiola at the dosage levels used in the clinical trials. Based on these intial studies in healthy adults, investigations into the usefulness of rhodiola in cases of CFS/FM seem rational. Supplementation with rhodiola has not been evaluated in pregnancy and lactation and should therefore be avoided during these times.

CHLORELLA PYRENOIDOSA

This single-cell green algae grows in fresh water; it is rich in protein (58 percent), chlorophyll, carotenoids, and a number of vitamins and minerals. There have been a number of animal studies showing that chlorella protects the intestinal lining, has anti-tumor properties, cholesterol-lowering properties, and can prevent the intestinal absorption of environmental toxins such as dioxin. The chlorophyll in chlorella has been shown to be the main component responsible for preventing dioxin absorption via foods. Chlorella has been shown in clinical trials to reduce the symptoms of fibromyalgia, inflammatory bowel disease, and hypertension.

Chlorella appears to have some positive health effects, but some caution needs to be exercised regarding overzealous marketing to FM patients. While it is true that chlorella has improved the symptoms of FM in both open-label and controlled studies, the doses used were so high they are beyond the financial means of virtually every FM patient. Be advised that the doses used in the FM studies involved fifty tablets and 100 ml of chlorella per day for two months—if you were to follow this regimen it would cost you about five hundred dollars a month.

It is unknown whether sustained low doses of chlorella, at levels found in green-food supplements, may have some therapeutic effect in CFS/FM over time. Based on the encouraging results of commercially available greens+ on energy, taking smaller doses combined with other antioxidant phytonutrients may be worthwhile. Chlorella is generally well tolerated; however, allergic reactions and photosensitivity have been reported after chlorella consumption. It should be avoided in pregnancy and nursing, and caution is advised in those on warfarin due to high vitamin K content.

LICORICE

Licorice, known botanically as *Glycyrrhiza glabra*, contains important antioxidant polyphenols. These protective chemicals in licorice have been shown to protect liver mitochondria (energy cells) against oxidative stress-related damage. Licorice has traditionally been used for adrenal gland support and is reported to improve cellular immune function in addition to its antiallergic, anti-ulcer, and anti-inflammatory properties. There is widespread use of licorice within traditional Asian herbal medicine, as it is said to enhance the usefulness of other herbs. The area of real interest regarding licorice and CFS is related to its ability to support adrenal gland function because the active component glycyrrhizin affects cortisol production and mimics the activity of the adrenal hormone aldosterone, which influences salt and water retention.

Former CFS patient and Italian physician Riccardo Baschetti has spent the last decade writing letters to medical journals in an effort to raise awareness of adrenal insufficiency in CFS and the value of licorice. When I looked on Medline, I found thirty letters to the editors of medical journals by Dr. Baschetti related to CFS adrenal function, licorice, or both. If nothing else, the guy is persistent. He recommends 2.5 g a day of licorice mixed in milk.

I highly recommend that all CFS/FM patients who supplement with licorice, particularly if following the protocol used by Dr. Baschetti, should do so under the supervision of an MD, DO, or licensed ND. Licorice supplementation is serious business and can cause rapid increases in blood pressure after less than two weeks of moderate use. Although all kinds of doses have been declared safe in the past, more recent research in the journal *Human and Experimental Toxicology* suggests that any glycyrrhizin level above 2 mg per kilogram of body weight (or 120 mg for a 132-pound person) has the potential for adverse effects (high blood pressure) in healthy adults. Many licorice products on the market are standardized to contain 22 percent glycyrrhizin, which means 1000 mg capsules will contain 220 mg of glycyrrhizin. Licorice products labelled DGL contain de-glycyrrhizinated licorice, in which the active glycyrrhizin has been completely or almost completely removed. DGL products are not associated with the adverse effects of standardized licorice, but neither will they exert any significant beneficial effect in adrenal support for CFS patients. DGL products are mainly promoted for healing the gastrointestinal lining.

There is a fairly solid theoretical background on the use of licorice in CFS; the available evidence suggests that licorice may help with the commonly reported low blood pressure on standing but that there is a fine line regarding dose. The antioxidant and liver protective properties are also potentially valuable. Patients I have interviewed generally report that licorice provides short-term improvement in symptoms, and it is generally well tolerated. However, more than a few patients report feeling revved up or "wired." The bottom line on licorice is that it may be helpful; however, it should be taken under a doctor's supervision.

ST. JOHN'S WORT

This well-known herbal antidepressant has received a significant amount of negative press over the last few years. Research has called into question the safety and efficacy of St. John's wort

(SJW). Despite two highly publicized U.S. trials, which showed SJW was no better than placebo, according to a recent review published in *European Archives of Psychiatry and Clinical Neuroscience*, the preponderance of evidence indicates that SJW can still be effective for mild to moderate depression. The media played up the fact that SJW was no better than placebo. They paid less attention to the fact that the little sugar pill performed as well as the active, and FDA approved, antidepressant drug sertraline (Zoloft)! The most recent, largest, and perhaps most well-designed trial showed that SJW is more effective than placebo for mild to moderate depression. Although the efficacy of SJW is similar to that of most antidepressants for non-severe depression, it is associated with far fewer side effects. SJW is generally well tolerated, with 2.4 percent of users reporting an adverse reaction. The most common adverse reactions include gastrointestinal discomfort, insomnia, and headaches. Although not commonly reported, skin may become hypersensitive to sun exposure after administration of SJW.

An area of real concern regarding SJW is co-administration with other drugs. SJW can speed up the elimination of medications from the body due to its effects on drug-metabolizing enzymes in the liver. There are a host of drugs that may be affected by SJW—about half of all marketed drugs, including blood-thinning medications and oral contraceptives. SJW should also not be co-administered with traditional antidepressant medications due to the risk of serotonin syndrome (too much serotonin).

The bottom line with SJW is that it may be effective in improving mild to moderate depression, and it has the added value of strong antioxidant activity. The antiviral activity of SJW gets promoted on various Web sites but human studies show no antiviral effect. The EPA concentrate from fish oil may enhance the effects of SJW; however, clinical supervision by an MD, DO, or licensed ND is highly recommended. Look for a product standardized to 3 to 6 percent hyperforin and 0.12 to 0.28 percent hypericin. The dose is typically 300 mg three times a day. However, make sure you discuss SJW and EPA with your doctor.

GINSENG

This is one of the most popular herbs for fatigue—ginseng, in its many forms, is often recommended to CFS/FM patients who visit the health food store. I would recommend CFS/FM patients avoid *Panax ginseng* due to its stimulatory effects and association with a collection of symptoms known as ginseng abuse syndrome—high blood pressure, agitation, sleeplessness, morning diarrhea, and skin eruptions. Siberian ginseng (*Eleutherococcus senticosus*) may be a more appropriate choice, but I would recommend that if taken it should be used at low doses (see below) and combined with the antioxidants discussed above. A small body of research supports the use of Siberian ginseng (SG) in humans under physical and emotional stress. SG seems to have a regulating effect on stress; it has been suggested through human and animal research that there is a threshold of stress below which SG increases the stress response and above which SG decreases the stress response. Experimental studies show that SG has antiviral and antiallergy properties, and like some other herbal ingredients, SG has known antioxidant activity. The data on SG are not particularly strong; the older Russian clinical data and the animal studies are intriguing, but they do not justify the sales hype as a solo supplement. Rhodiola appears to have more potential in treating CFS/FM.

CFS/FM patients should stay below 100 mg of ginseng a day; at this level there are no well-documented adverse effects. Despite what you may see on the Internet and in some books, there is no research showing that after one to two months of use, SG needs to be discontinued for two weeks in order to be effective. Some plant-based nutrient products, such as greens+, combine low levels of herbal antioxidants such as SG, ginkgo, etc.

SUMMARY

- Supplements are not a substitute for a healthy, nutritious diet.
- Some nutritional and herbal supplements have therapeutic potential in CFS/FM, however, numerous supplements offer false hope.
- Harvard researchers suggested in 2002 that all North American adults take a multivitamin every day. Think of a multi as a dietary insurance policy.
- Essential fatty acids from the omega-3 family are currently underconsumed in North America. Limited data suggests that omega-3 fatty acids from fish oil, particularly EPA, may be beneficial in CFS, FM, and depression. Research shows only 1 g of EPA is required to improve treatment-resistant depression. EPA is a potent anti-inflammatory fatty acid. Concentrated EPA is now available in the United States and Canada as o3mega+ joy™.
- Specific strains of probiotics (beneficial bacteria) have potential to improve a number of CFS/FM symptoms, in the gut and beyond. Only a few probiotic stains on the market have peer-reviewed research to support physiologi-

---

What's in greens+?

Phosphatide complex (phosphatidyl choline from lecithin)	Royal jelly
Organic alfalfa, barley, wheat grass, and red beet powder	Bee pollen
	Full spectrum grape extract
Spirulina	Licorice root extract
Apple pectin	Acerola berry juice powder
Japanese Chlorella	Siberian ginseng extract
Organic soy sprouts	Milk thistle extract
Organic whole brown rice powder	Organic Nova Scotia dulse powder
Stevia leaf powder	Ginkgo biloba extract
Non-dairy bacterial cultures containing *Lactobacilli* and *Bifidobacteria*	Japanese green tea extract
	European bilberry extract

cal activity. *Lactobacillus* GG and *Lactobacillus casei* strain Shirota (Yakult) are among the few strains with documented activity and therapeutic potential in CFS/FM and related symptoms.

- Calcium, magnesium, folic acid, and vitamin B12 are important dietary and supplemental considerations for CFS/FM patients. Calcium is essential in the prevention of osteoporosis in CFS/FM patients.

- SAMe, 5-HTP, and melatonin may be of limited value in CFS/FM.

- Chlorella, rhodiola, St. John's wort, and licorice may have therapeutic potential, but a doctor should supervise when supplementing.

- Recent research on a powdered food product, greens+, has shown that it can increase energy in adults.

- Supplements and the term "natural" are not to be translated as "safe." They are not immune from negative physiological effects and potential interactions with prescription drugs.

HERMAN®

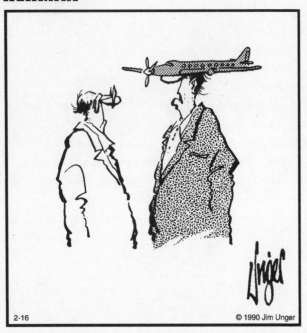

2-16

"I've decided to expand my horizons."

CHAPTER SIX

MIND-BODY MEDICINE

Modern scientific research and the use of a placebo in drug trials have proven that the mind and body are not separate and distinct from each other. It is estimated that over 35 percent of subjects in clinical trials report significant improvements due to placebo (sugar pill) response. The significance of this is currently under-appreciated in modern medicine—often dismissed as non-treatment. In fact, the so-called "placebo response" is far from non-treatment; it is actually a very powerful medicine. According to research published in *Biological Psychiatry*, the placebo is able to match almost 80 percent of an antidepressant drug effect over extended periods of time.

Thankfully, modern brain imaging techniques have shown that those who truly *believe* they are taking a powerful drug (even if they are actually taking a sugar pill) can change their brain chemistry. In a study published in the *American Journal of Psychiatry* in 2002, researchers from the University of Toronto showed that the placebo was able to induce changes in brain glucose metabolism in alleviating depression. Although not surprising to those who have been researching the effects of the placebo, these results are groundbreaking. Additional research published in the *New England Journal of Medicine* in 2002 showed that actual knee surgery for osteoarthritis was not better than "sham" or simulated surgery in reducing pain over a two-year period. In addition, researchers from the UCLA Department of Psychiatry showed that changing thoughts and behavioral patterns can, without using drugs, positively alter the brain chemistry of those with obsessive-compulsive disorder. These are just a few examples; there are more than two thousand studies in well-respected medical journals substantiating the value of mind-body medicine.

Understanding that the mind and the body are not separate entities is extremely important in your recovery efforts. While mind-body therapies are not a cure-all, nor are they a substitute for appropriate medical care, they have the potential to alter the course of CFS/FM in a positive way. In dealing with a life-

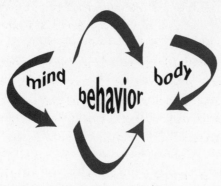

Mind, body, and behavior can all influence each other.

altering illness, CFS/FM patients need to do what they can to gain some sense of control over the illness and develop coping skills. The therapies that comprise mind-body medicine can do just that.

WHAT IS MIND-BODY MEDICINE?

Mind-body medicine is a broad term for a number of techniques/therapies that take full consideration of the mind (thoughts and emotions) and its ability to alter health status and, by the same token, fully consider the disordered body and its influence on the mind. Simply put, the mind and body are one. These techniques and therapies include, but are not limited to, meditation (including mindfulness and the relaxation response), hypnotherapy, biofeedback, guided imagery/visualization, yoga, prayer, tai chi, breathing exercises, therapeutic writing/art, and, importantly, cognitive-behavioral therapy. Basically it is a buffet of therapies with no limit on your choices, and while not every therapy will work for every person, most patients benefit from at least one of these techniques. The real beauty of mind-body medicine is the relatively low cost of the various therapies.

In our research presented at the Sixth International Conference on CFS, FM and Related Illnesses in February 2003 in Washington, D.C., Dr. Bested and I found that more than 90 percent of 134 CFS patients (sample, metro Toronto) were performing some type of mind-body technique on a regular basis. Of those using mind-body interventions, meditation was the most frequently reported, followed by breathing exercises, stretching, prayer, imagery/visualization, and yoga. Of those using mind-body therapies, approximately half reported them to be very helpful or somewhat helpful in managing the symptoms of CFS. It seems that CFS patients are pretty happy with mind-body medicine. FM patients have also been shown to respond well to mind-body medicine; research published in the *Journal of Rheumatology* indicates that mind-body therapies are as valuable as many current treatment approaches. Let's take a closer look.

MEDITATION

The origins of meditation, dating back some three thousand years, are traced to the Indian subcontinent. Although there are numerous meditation techniques, I will focus on the two main categories—mindfulness and concentration.

As pointed out in a recent article in the journal *American Family Physician*, mindfulness meditation may be particularly valuable in FM, and I would suggest that it might be just as important in those with CFS. The reason is that in the practice of mindfulness, a CFS/FM patient is neither in the past nor the future—only in the here and now. There is much to be said for that: focus on the now, the present, is not associated with frightening "what if" future thinking, the negative experiences of the past, or contemplation of the good times when life was not enveloped in pain and fatigue. It's a time to simply be—a moment of acceptance, an awareness of life. Mindfulness meditation is, however, a time to feel and take stock of emotions, to not force them away, a process that may not always be comfortable, but one that can be normal and natural. Mindfulness doesn't require a particular position or location; you don't even need an expensive "as seen on TV, limited edition" mat to sit on! You can practice mindfulness meditation in its simplest form by taking a walk and observing your environment—the intricate details of leaves, the texture of wood or sand. Pick up a raisin or a walnut—have you ever really looked at the fine details before you chow down? Mindfulness is awareness, patience, inquiry, and, ultimately, insight.

Concentration meditation requires undivided attention on a designated object; it may be an image, word, sound (mantra), or the physical sensation and experience of the breath itself. While this does require a level of concentration that may be difficult for some CFS/FM patients, the benefits are derived from what is actually being excluded: the worries, stressors, and everyday "stuff" that can make our minds so unnecessarily busy. When distractions arise, such as external sounds and intrusive thoughts, simply return to the object of focus and continue the meditation. I say "simply," but I understand that it can be difficult. However, with practice and a little persistence, this can become incorporated into your daily routine. I have discussed the value of meditation with many CFS/FM patients, and the majority have been impressed by the payoff of taking a little time out. In the case of FM, mediation has been shown to be a valuable tool in the management of the illness.

Dr. Herbert Benson of Harvard Medical School, a pioneer in mind-body medicine, has determined (based on years of scientific research) the following regarding his form of concentration meditation called the *relaxation response*.

1. Best performed in a quiet, comfortable environment, in a comfortable position.
2. Consciously relax the muscles of the body.
3. Repeat a simple mental stimulus such as a word, phrase, image, or prayer.
4. Adopt a passive mental attitude toward the process itself and any intrusions.
5. Perform this relaxation response for ten to twenty minutes.

The name *relaxation response* comes from the physiological

Table 1. Physiological effects of the stress response and the autonomic nervous system. The use of the relaxation response can diminish the negative effects of chronic sympathetic dominance.

PARASYMPATHETIC	SYMPATHETIC
Rest and digest	Alarm
Heart rate/force decreased	Heart rate/force increased
Digestion increased	Digestion slowed
Adrenal output decreased	Adrenal glands stressed
Protection from foreign particles	Decreased saliva/mucus
Conservation of energy	Energy consumption
Elimination of waste	Waste not removed

effects of performing the above steps. In simple terms, the relaxation response is the opposite of the *stress response* or the "fight or flight" response. Under stress, the body will respond by domination of the sympathetic nervous system, which causes an increase in the levels of the hormones epinephrine and norepinephrine and a host of physiological effects (Table 1) that are appropriate in the short term but devastating to health over the long term. When one engages the relaxation response, there are natural physiological consequences as well. However, in contrast to the stress response, these changes are associated with good health. The relaxation response can dampen a sympathetic dominance and allow for activity of the parasympathetic branch of the autonomic nervous system. Research conducted by Dr. Benson (or by colleagues who have examined the relaxation response) indicates that it is helpful in a wide variety of medical conditions.

I have taken close to one hundred hours of continuing education and clinical training in mind-body medicine under the direction of Dr. Benson at Harvard Medical School. In addition, I had the good fortune to be invited to attend Harvard's Mind-Body Institute's specific training in the chronic fatigue syndrome/chronic pain specialty clinic. I still feel honored to be the first naturopathic physician to be granted this privilege. Harvard's specialty clinic designed for the treatment of chronic fatigue syndrome/chronic pain makes a positive and very significant impact on the patients who experience these conditions. The focus is on:

- Teaching coping skills
- Changing perceptions and negative thought processes
- Eliciting the relaxation response and choosing from the mind-body buffet
- Exercise within limitations
- Humor and optimism
- Effective problem solving
- Establishing a non-toxic social support system
- Setting realistic goals
- Gaining control over the things that can be controlled and letting go of those things we cannot control
- Establishing a commitment to wellness, even though it is a gradual process for CFS/FM patients
- Expression of emotion, including therapeutic writing
- Healthy nutrition

Patients who live in the New England area should take advantage of this program if circumstances permit; others should seek out direct affiliate programs or those that are modeled after the Harvard program, such as Dr. Bested's in Toronto. Let's continue our look at the mind-body buffet.

BREATHING EXERCISES

Breathing techniques to induce relaxation are part of a number of mind-body modalities, including meditation and yoga. There are a variety of different techniques, but perhaps abdominal breathing is most well known. Abdominal breathing was known in the past as diaphragmatic breathing, but today we know that the diaphragm is involved in all normal breathing. The diaphragm is a sheet of muscle attached to the lower ribs and in a relaxed state looks like a dome. When it contracts, the dome flattens out and causes the abdominal area to enlarge. When engaging in abdominal breathing, you should be in a comfortable position, breathing at a natural pace (probably more slowly than usual) with a focus on the abdomen swelling downwards with each breath in. Place your hand over your abdomen while getting comfortable with the process. Your hand should sink in toward your body on the out breath. This abdominal breathing is in contrast to stressful breathing, which has a greater emphasis on the upper ribs and use of shoulder muscles. Becoming more aware of your breathing and teaching yourself to breathe at a normal pace may prevent hyperventilation syndrome, associated with taking too many shallow breaths. Interestingly, hyperventilation syndrome shares some CFS/FM signs and symptoms, including reduced blood flow to the brain, dizziness, headaches, visual disturbances, and panic attacks.

COGNITIVE-BEHAVIORAL THERAPY

While some over-enthusiastic scientists and practitioners view cognitive-behavioral therapy (CBT) as the *only* treatment of value in CFS/FM recovery efforts (much to the chagrin of patient advocacy groups), there can be no doubt about its powerful effects in helping patients learn to deal with life-altering chronic illness. The cognitive portion of the therapy is designed to identify and address negative thoughts and beliefs. In living with a chronic illness, it is important to understand that certain thoughts and beliefs can have a negative effect on not only mood but also on physical health and ultimately behavior. Cognitive distortions or so-called "faulty thinking" patterns are those that eliminate the positive, over-exaggerate the negative, and involve a lot of "what if" future thinking—and those thoughts are not productive ones like "what if things go really well?" or "what if they do understand that I have a chronic illness?" In any chronic condition, certain negative thoughts, images, and beliefs can interfere with the recovery effort and diminish hope and overall quality of life. That negative thoughts arise in states of chronic illness is normal and natural—after all, chronic illness impacts on virtually every aspect of life. CFS/FM patients report losing "friends," feeling less valuable, and being unable to function in many aspects, yet feeling guilty for it and at the same time wondering how many people are thinking they are just lazy, malingering, or have some strange, contagious disease. These are difficult issues, particularly because the vast majority of patients were very high-functioning individuals before their illness. Reshaping how you approach these (any many other) issues in your thoughts and beliefs can be a major step toward coping—a key word in your recovery plan. It may also, according to the scientific research, have a positive effect on your body's physiology.

The behavioral portion of therapy will examine closely your energy expenditure/physical activity to help you identify when you may be overdoing it and help identify triggers that worsen symptoms. Physical activity is important in recovery efforts but must be undertaken in a most delicate fashion. Dr. Bested uses an activity log with all patients to access energy/pain levels and associations with physical activity. From this, patients learn to pace themselves, maintain physical activity, and sort out the actions that may contribute to flare-ups. Patients learn to think of their body as a battery with a certain amount of energy inside. They are encouraged to use most of that energy on a given day but not to go into reserves that are unavailable, as is the case when problems arise. On days when a patient wakes up feeling more pro-

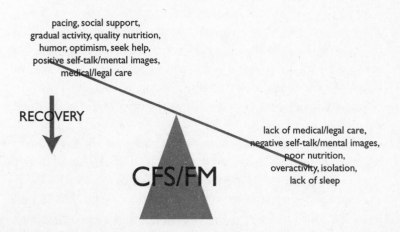

pacing, social support, gradual activity, quality nutrition, humor, optimism, seek help, positive self-talk/mental images, medical/legal care

RECOVERY

CFS/FM

lack of medical/legal care, negative self-talk/mental images, poor nutrition, overactivity, isolation, lack of sleep nounced fatigue/pain, these are days to conserve energy or recharge the battery.

There is no shortage of research documenting the wonderful effects of CBT, not only in CFS/FM but in a host of chronic illnesses, most notably within the realm of classic mental health (anxiety and depression) and in so-called functional syndromes such as irritable bowel and chronic headaches. However, CBT has also proven itself useful in illnesses with more clearly described physiological abnormalities, including arthritis, diabetes, cardiovascular disease, and chronic pain. That CBT would be effective in improving the symptoms and/or the quality of life of those with these and other conditions, once again, shows that the line between mind and body is not distinct.

Despite the benefits of CBT, it is important to point out that the "faulty thinking and actions" (those to be corrected by CBT) did *not* cause your CFS or FM. Simply put, the onset of CFS/FM is not your fault, and don't ever let anyone tell you otherwise. It also must be stressed that the benefits of CBT are in addressing the chronic illness and the application of the therapy is not unique to CFS/FM. Yes, there is research showing that many CFS/FM patients were very high energy before illness onset, perhaps lacking the ability to say no to physical and emotional demands. Sure, there is research showing that many CFS/FM patients had significant emotional and physical stressors before illness onset. However, there really isn't anything unique about this. There are countless illnesses connected to stress, even the common cold. If faulty thinking and actions were the cause of CFS/FM or if stress were the *direct and only* cause of these illnesses, then millions more North Americans would have these conditions.

After years of running from doctor to doctor and undergoing test after test without a proper diagnosis, it is understandable that many CFS/FM patients are reluctant to get involved with CBT. Patients have already been told one too many times that "it's all in your head," and the research showing that there are indeed physiological abnormalities in CFS/FM seems to be discounted or ignored completely by many. However, patients who pursue CBT are not acknowledging that CFS/FM are psychological conditions; they are simply exploring a potentially therapeutic treatment option. Many patients I have interviewed described the experience of CBT as a turning point in recovery efforts. One thing is sure: the conditions of CFS/FM leave the patient with a diminished ability to handle stress, and this is an important area where CBT can be helpful. In her integrative clinic in Toronto, Dr. Bested hosts CBT groups for CFS/FM patients under the direction of Jack Birnbaum, psychiatrist and Canadian CBT expert. I would encourage all CFS/FM patients to seek out and work in collaboration with a qualified mental health professional in order to take advantage of the benefits of CBT.

PRAYER AND RELIGION

Patients with chronic illnesses often pray and are prayed for, and many report using religious beliefs as a means of coping with illness. Modern scientific studies have looked at in-person prayer and intercessory prayer where the patient does not know he or she is being prayed for. Findings indicate that such prayers have potential value in a number of medical conditions, including cardiovascular disease, arthritis, infertility, blood infections, anxiety, and psychological well-being. Researchers have also investigated the influence of religious activities and found that they are associated with many positive health parameters, including immune function, regulation of blood pressure, improved mood, and decreased mortality. These beneficial findings are not specific to any one of the major religions or sects; they are related to comforting beliefs and the social support that religion can provide. Dr. Harold Koenig of Duke University is a leading expert on religion and medicine; he reports that religiosity provides hope, control, strength, meaning, and purpose to those with medical conditions.

BIOFEEDBACK

The modality of biofeedback takes advantage of the fact that human beings can, to a certain point, influence parts of physiology that were once thought to be under strict unconscious control. A practitioner of biofeedback can teach patients, with the aid of various auditory or visual devices, how to obtain some conscious control over a variety of bodily functions. The devices are often technology-based, including EEG machines that can measure brain waves. A very simple form of biofeedback is called the biodot, a small skin-temperature-sensitive disc that is placed on the web of the thumb and first finger. When an individual is in a relaxed state, there is increased blood flow to the extremities and the disc changes color. Dr. Bested uses these biodots in group sessions, and she finds that patients love them as a basic guide as they practice the relaxation response. Biofeedback training can be a means to reduce CFS/FM symptoms such as muscle tension, headaches, and gastrointestinal complaints. One case report in the journal *Behavioral Medicine* indicates that biofeedback may be helpful for the cognitive difficulties in CFS (or perhaps the "fibrofog" decribed by FM patients). See the Appendix for more information on biodots as a means of measuring blood flow and relaxation.

HYPNOTHERAPY

Medical hypnosis is a technique that involves suggestion, by a therapist, that a patient experience changes in perception, thought, sensation, and behavior. It is a voluntary state of selective focus which has been described as somewhere between sleep and wakefulness. Through the induction of deep relaxation, the patient is able to concentrate, use imagery, and be open to suggestions (goal-oriented instruction) that may positively influence health and behavior. Medical hypnotherapy is not a circus act with a watch on a chain. It has been the subject of much scientific research, with studies showing its ability to help with various medical conditions and symptoms, including gastrointestinal disorders, skin conditions, headaches, chronic pain, and anxiety. In the case of FM, a study published in the *Journal of Rheumatology* compared hypnotherapy to physical therapy and showed that those in the hypnotherapy group had greater reductions in pain, fatigue, and sleep problems. Hypnotherapy should be considered a potential therapeutic option as a means to reduce the symptoms of CFS/FM.

GUIDED IMAGERY

Mental imagery is defined as an experience that is similar to a perceptual event but is distinguished by the absence of stimuli. Having a picnic lunch on top of a hill overlooking beautiful fields of green and a rolling brook with the sounds and smells of summer involves *actual* perceptions of visual, auditory, olfactory (smell), taste, touch, and temperature stimuli. The human brain has an amazing ability to generate images of this scene, even if the "visualizer" is in a high-rise condominium during a freezing day in a Toronto winter—i.e., in the absence of stimuli. If I asked you to visualize cutting a fresh lemon into quarters, visualize the bitter juices flowing from the lemon as you squeeze it into a glass, such images may provoke salivation in your mouth.

Most of the anxiety we experience in our lives is a result of negative future thinking and visualizing negative images. Negative imagery brings about negative physiological responses; merely visualizing an upcoming stressful event can lead to racing heart, upset stomach, and other changes associated with the stress response. We can, however, turn these negative images around for health promotion and improved performance. Guided imagery, as taught by mental health professionals, involves the use of positive imagery and has been found to be useful in a host of medical conditions including chronic pain, headaches, multiple sclerosis, anxiety, and overall stress reduction. Imagery has been found to be particularly useful in hospital settings, where it is used as a means of pain management. Imagery can be combined with music therapy, which has benefits in its own right.

Guided imagery has recently been studied in FM with a very favorable outcome. A study published in the *Journal of Psychiatric Research* showed that pleasant imagery (vs. attention imagery and no-imagery control groups) was effective in reducing FM pain during the one-month study. Pleasant guided imagery involved visualization of beautiful, natural summertime settings, while the attention imagery group visualized physiological events related to pain control such as release of the pain-reducing chemical endorphin and nervous system cells that can inhibit pain. FM patients, it seems, need to focus away from pain altogether in visualization exercises. When CFS/FM patients acquire a comfortable level of skill and experience, then self-guided imagery can take over where the outside practitioner left off. There are very useful audiotapes available to help with such visualization and the transition to self-guided imagery.

YOGA/TAI CHI

Yoga and tai chi are modalities that capture the essence of mind-body medicine because they both incorporate physical movement with the emotional being. They are particularly effective for CFS/FM patients because in contrast to Western-style exercise, yoga and tai chi are associated with less impact and extreme physical exertion (therefore they induce less post-exertional fatigue and pain). Although yoga and tai chi can certainly be physically and mentally challenging, both modalities can be adapted, modified, and individually tailored for CFS/FM patients.

Hatha yoga is one of the more well-known forms of yoga in Western culture; it is based on an awareness of and a balance between both psychological and physical energies. In Hatha yoga, it is the breath that is the essential component in the union of mind and body; through proper breathing control, one can absorb the life force or *prana*. Research into Hatha yoga as a medical intervention shows that it can reduce pain and increase range of motion in osteoarthritis, improve grip strength and reduce pain in carpal tunnel syndrome, improve cardiovascular and lung function, and improve oxygen delivery to body tissue.

Tai chi combines physical movement, meditation, and breathing. The usual outcome is relaxation of the mind, improved balance, coordination, and conditioning. In tai chi there is a focus on abdominal breathing in coordination with movement. It is proper abdominal breathing that is thought to enhance the flow of energy or *qi* (pronounced *chee*) throughout the body. As with yoga, there are numerous different postures and styles, a number of which may not be appropriate for CFS/FM. Modifications, including a lying-down position and the support of pillows, may be necessary. In general, CFS/FM patients can tolerate most tai chi movements quite well and may find improvements not only in relative endurance, strength, flexibility, and balance but, importantly, in emotional well-being as well. Recent research has shown tai chi can lead to improvement in cardiorespiratory function, balance and postural stability, fall prevention, and overall stress reduction.

It is important in CFS/FM recovery efforts to find some sort of satisfying physical activity plan that can be performed within the limitations of the individual. To get started, it is best to see a trained yoga or tai chi instructor who will help you with a modified plan.

THERAPEUTIC WRITING/ART

Confronting difficult life experiences through writing and art can have very positive effects on both emotional and physical well-being. Dr. James Pennebaker has shown in published research that those who write about traumatic life events as opposed to superficial topics show subsequent (although not immediate) improvements in mood and decreased use of health care services. In addition, individuals who write about the facts and the emotions surrounding stressful events in life show heightened immune function versus those who only write about the facts. There are more than a dozen studies demonstrating that writing about stressful or traumatic events can improve various health-related outcomes, including improvements in symptoms of arthritis and asthma.

The pen and paper discussion should involve expression of your deepest emotions, including what you feel and why you feel it. Writing about events that seem to be constantly on your mind is most appropriate; you can be the one who defines "traumatic." For many patients with CFS/FM, it may be how the illness has turned their lives upside down, or more specifically, it may be about now-changed personal relationships or physical and professional limitations—it's really for you to decide. Write as if it's just for you; don't plan on sharing your writing with anyone at all; this way you will be less likely to hold anything back out of fear of embarrassment or punishment. You can, if you like, dispose of the writings after you are finished if you are concerned about others reading very personal material.

Artwork is also a form of emotional expression. In Dr. Bested's education and support group, during week two, all patients draw/illustrate what their life is like now as they deal with CFS/FM. They are also asked to draw, separately, what life would be like in a state of recovery from CFS/FM. These exercises and the images that result are incredibly moving—despite the emotional difficulty and the frequent tears, virtually all patients report that it is a wonderful and worthwhile experience. Patients report a sense of relief when they complete the "now" drawing and a sense of hope and optimism when they complete the "recovery" piece.

An additional form of art that may be very worthwhile is reciting some old-fashioned poetry. Research published in the *International Journal of Cardiology* shows that when subjects recite poetic (rhythmic) verse while walking and breathing in time to the "beat" of the poem, there is a reduction in heart rate and an increase in vagal (vagus nerve) tone. Low vagal tone may be an indicator of stress vulnerability, and interestingly, vagal tone is decreased in CFS patients. This type of art therapy, recitation while walking, is a true mind-body therapy where, once again, breath may be the important link. Rhythm (not necessarily rhyme) is crucial, as it synchronizes breath with heartbeat.

Therapeutic writing and art should be a part of the CFS/FM recovery efforts. Research supports its effects on mood, cardiovascular function, and the immune system—so why not give it a try?

ADDITIONAL NOTES

Dr. Suzanne Kobasa of the City University of New York has identified three defining characteristics of so-called "stress-hardiness"; they are the three Cs: *commitment*, *control*, and *challenge*. Individuals who possess the three Cs appear to have a degree of immunity to the devastating effects of stress—they are immersed in what they are doing, committed to the end, they believe they are in control and that they can influence outcomes, and they see change as a challenge.

There is no evidence to show that "stress-hardy" people are immune from CFS and FM; of course they are not. However, we shouldn't dismiss the three Cs; the research shows that CFS/FM patients are more vulnerable to stress *after* illness onset, so patients should do everything they possibly can to minimize the effects of stress. Perhaps the three Cs may help in dealing with stressors as you proceed on your journey toward recovery. Despite the waxing and waning of symptoms, the chronic nature of the illnesses, and its effects on your personal and professional lives, do everything you can to stay committed to recovery, to believe that you can influence the outcome (through appropriate medical care, nutrition, rest, physical activity, and available treatments), and to view recovery as personal growth and development.

CHAPTER SUMMARY

- The human mind and body are not separate. Research on the placebo effect indicates just how powerful belief can be in human health and physiology.

- Mind-body medicine includes various techniques/therapies that consider the mind (thoughts and emotions) and its influence on the body—and the disordered body and its influence on the mind.
- Research indicates that CFS/FM patients often use mind-body therapies and they are at least somewhat helpful.
- Mind-body therapies are not a cure, nor are they a substitute for appropriate medical intervention. They can, however, help patients to cope with chronic illness and are a cost-effective means of symptom reduction.

CHAPTER SEVEN

COMPLEMENTARY THERAPIES

The term *complementary and alternative medicine* (CAM) refers to a broad range of healing modalities that are generally not taught in medical schools and are not available in most North American hospitals. There is often a lack of middle ground among medical professionals with regard to attitudes toward CAM; there is either unbridled enthusiasm or vehement opposition. This is often reflected in books on CFS/FM where some discount CAM modalities as useless and a waste of time and money, while others will promise that various devices and gadgets, diets, pills, and potions can help cure CFS/FM.

There is a middle ground to be found; perhaps some of the modalities within CAM may be therapeutically valuable. Dr. Bested has recognized this. She has not thrown away the wonderful tools of orthodox medicine, nor has she discontinued using prescription medications that can make a tremendous difference in the life of patients, but rather she has remained open-minded and integrated CAM therapies when they have been shown to be helpful. This is what integrative medicine is all about—utilizing the best of both orthodox and CAM approaches. It is important to point out that CAM should never be a substitute for proper medical treatment. The purpose of this chapter is to provide a brief overview of major CAM modalities and discuss their place in the treatment of CFS/FM. I will discuss some of the individual CAM modalities below, but first a little background on CAM in North America.

North Americans turn to CAM in high numbers when they have chronic illnesses, particularly those such as CFS/FM, irritable bowel syndrome, multiple chemical sensitivities, and others that remain medically unexplained. These conditions involve a myriad of symptoms, and when an MD is faced with such a mixed bag of chronic symptoms that seem treatment resistant, it can be overwhelming. Physicians often begin to see psychology in the conditions and not physiology. When a syndrome is medically unexplained and there are no medications that can help cure the illness, conditions are ripe for patients to explore CAM therapies.

The average span of time between onset of symptoms and actually getting a diagnosis of CFS/FM is five to seven years, so they tend to bounce around from family doctors to specialists.

Sometimes it can be the attitude of the treating physician that is the most significant factor in turning a patient toward CAM. One patient I interviewed had waited for a couple of months for a referral with a rheumatologist to query FM. At the visit, the rheumatologist introduced himself, and the patient began describing her widespread muscular pain, at which point the doctor cut her off and said, "You don't look like you are in any pain." This interaction subsequently led to a visit to a CAM practitioner for help. This anecdote is not a knock on rheumatologists in general—there are thousands out there helping FM patients in their recovery efforts with a limited arsenal of treatments. Sadly, though, there are too many stories like this one,

HERMAN®

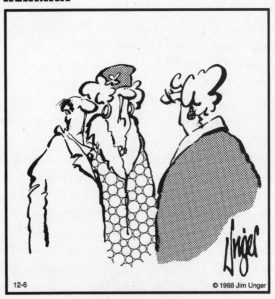

12-6   © 1988 Jim Unger

**"He thinks a chiropractor is an
Egyptian doctor."**

because there are far too many physicians who just don't buy into CFS/FM as physical illnesses. The MDs and DOs who understand CFS/FM and what is known about their physiological effects are brave individuals who deserve the utmost respect. I have seen Dr. Bested and other like-minded colleagues give lectures on CFS/FM to mainstream doctors, only to be met with resistance and dismissal. The attitudes of doctors toward CFS/FM are very much like the massive division in attitudes toward CAM.

Research shows that up to 80 percent of North Americans and Europeans who use CAM modalities are satisfied with them, while only 40 percent report satisfaction with orthodox, science-based approaches. Those who use CAM report it to be more empowering and more individualistic. The majority (two out of three) of CFS/FM patients have reported that they are dissatisfied with their quality of orthodox medical care, and many turn to CAM for help. The minority of patients who are satisfied with medical care perceive doctors to be caring, supportive, and inter-ested, and they evaluate "good" doctors not so much on their ability to treat CFS/FM but more on their interpersonal and informational skills. Research shows that only a very small group of patients will utilize CAM instead of standard orthodox care; the vast majority use both. Patients still appear reluctant to tell doctors of CAM use because they fear the doctor will judge them, or they feel it is unimportant. A few CFS patients I have inter-viewed report that family doctors have told them that they can-not continue being a patient if they are also seeking care from CAM providers. This is unfortunate, and it suggests that perhaps there is some validity to the patients' fear of CAM disclosure.

I would recommend finding a new GP/family doc if this is the unsupportive attitude you encounter. It is important that you feel supported in *your* health care choices; the goal should be to work together with your physician to improve your health. I would fur-ther recommend that you always disclose your use of CAM ther-apies and supplements to your doctor in the interest of safety.

One major reason for the sense of satisfaction with CAM is

likely related to time. The modern medical system is set up in such a way that MDs and DOs just do not have the luxury of time with patients, whereas CAM practitioners, other than chiropractors, spend much more time with patients. Research shows that MDs and chiropractors average about five to fifteen minutes with a patient, while naturopathic physicians (NDs) spend about forty minutes and massage therapists and acupuncturists spend about an hour. Patients interpret extended sessions as extended care. The luxury of time enhances the patient-practitioner relationship and allows the patient to deal with concerns that will not otherwise come up in the shorter visit.

CFS/FM patients are not alone in using CAM approaches; in 1997, more than 40 percent of Americans reported CAM use, with 629 million visits to CAM practitioners at an expense of 27 billion dollars! For perspective, consider that Americans made 386 million visits to GPs/primary care physicians and spent 29 billion dollars on physician-related medical care. That means more visits were made to CAM practitioners and more money was spent out of pocket on CAM practitioners. Patients with chronic illnesses, including CFS/FM, are two to three times more likely to see a CAM practitioner than their healthy counterparts.

What are these CAM modalities, and how useful are they in treating CFS/FM? The following is a discussion of some of the CAM therapies along with some important caveats that CFS/FM patients should know about. Herbal medicine is excluded; herbs that are reported to have specific value are discussed in the dietary and herbal supplements chapter. In general, herbs should be taken under the supervision of an MD, DO, or ND. You may find the following a little conservative, but I make no apologies for looking to science as a means to sort out CAM.

NATUROPATHIC MEDICINE

Let's start with this because I am a licensed naturopathic physician. It is my slightly biased opinion that naturopathic doctors (NDs) are best suited to bridge the gap between complementary and mainstream care. I say this because NDs are the only practitioners with graduate-level education in multiple CAM modalities; basically NDs are the general practitioners of CAM. To call yourself a licensed ND in the states (and provinces) that regulate the practice, you must complete the same pre-med classes as in orthodox medical school and four years of full-time graduate training in the basic medical sciences and the modalities of:

- Clinical nutrition
- Botanical medicine
- Acupuncture
- Homeopathy
- Hydrotherapy
- Counseling (including mind-body medicine)
- Physical medicine

In addition, licensure requires over twelve hundred hours of clinical supervision, passing of basic science and clinical board exams, as well as other requirements established by the states (and provinces).

The bottom line is that it is a rigorous program, and there are only five schools in North America that are accredited to grant doctor of naturopathic medicine degrees. There are, however, countless mail-order programs where so-called "graduates" can call themselves ND, PhD. Imagine granting an MD or a PhD in clinical psychology, a master's in social work, a nursing degree, or the registered dietician (RD) credentials through the mail without any supervised clinical experience! It would be preposterous, an outrage, yet that's exactly what goes on every day in the majority of states that don't have regulations for licensing of NDs. For this reason, if you live outside a licensed jurisdiction, it is essential that you inquire about the training of an ND before a visit.

The six principles of naturopathic medicine are identified in Table 1. In their efforts to promote wellness, NDs employ the treatment modalities listed above. In particular, clinical nutrition

Table 1.

Naturopathic medicine is not defined by a specific modality, as is acupuncture or chiropractic; it encompasses a number of complementary modalities and is officially defined by its six unifying principles.

1. **The Healing Power of Nature**
   We can witness the natural healing process when a cut heals in an orderly and intelligent fashion. NDs support and facilitate the healing process by aiding in the establishment of a healthy internal and external environment. Diet, lifestyle factors, and pacing are all examples of ways to facilitate the healing process in CFS/FM.

2. **Identify and Treat the Cause**
   Illness does not occur without cause(s). With complex, multifactoral illnesses such as CFS/FM, a cause or causes remain a mystery. As science continues to unravel the causes, NDs will address what is known and make appropriate recommendations to address the roots, not merely suppress the branches (symptoms). NDs practice in a holistic fashion where all possible contributing causes are considered in the context of an individual person. Physical, psychological, social, and environmental contributing factors are considered in attempting to identify the roots.

3. **First Do No Harm**
   NDs are mandated to use methods of treatment and medicinal substances that serve to minimize the risk of harmful effects.

4. **Doctor as Teacher**
   The word *doctor* translates as "teacher," and in fact NDs are expected to be teachers of health. The primary role of an ND is to empower patients to play a role in their own health care. This relationship maximizes the therapeutic potential of the doctor-patient relationship.

5. **Treat the Whole Person**
   The physiological alterations are experienced by each patient in an individual way, with genetic, emotional, social, psychological, and various environmental differences. NDs consider all of these complexities and understand that the *multifactorial* nature of health and disease requires an individualized approach that considers the whole body and mind as one.

6. **Prevention**
   Through education and the promotion of a healthy lifestyle, NDs consider prevention the primary goal of the profession. Unhealthy environment, susceptibilities, lifestyle, and various risk factors can breed illness; NDs consider this in promoting wellness. Prevention is important for CFS/FM patients; clearly, patients are not immune from developing other serious medical conditions.

is considered to be the cornerstone of naturopathic medicine, and the 220-plus hours of classroom training, in addition to supervised clinical experience (1,200 hours) and passage of national board exams in nutrition, ensures high standards. The same is true of the other modalities: 220-plus classroom hours of botanical medicine, supervised clinical experience, and passage of national board exams. I bring up these numbers because there are so many individuals and medical practitioners who hold themselves out as CAM "experts" yet have minimal training. When it comes to clinical nutrition, botanical medicine, and homeopathy, NDs are at a tremendous academic advantage.

Naturopathic doctors have been promoting a healthy lifestyle for years, long before it was in vogue to do so. They have been promoting healthy diets, omega-3 essential fatty acids, relaxation techniques, moderate exercise, liberal consumption of fruits and vegetables, etc., all of which have been validated by modern science. A good ND will incorporate many areas of research in order to set up an appropriate lifestyle plan to help improve your CFS/FM. Notice that I said *help*, not cure. If an ND promises a total cure, you will have to abandon Dr. Bested's pacing and energy conservation plan, and at that point I urge you to *run* from the office. Sad to say, they are out there, so beware.

Risks/Caveats

Holding a license means that an ND has devoted the time, energy, and expense necessary to fulfill the requirements set by lawmakers. However, being licensed does not automatically translate into being an effective clinician. Based on my interviews with CFS/FM patients, there are a couple of issues you should be aware of regarding NDs and treatment.

First is the over-prescribing of dietary supplements and herbal products. A minority of NDs suggest far, far too many supplements for CFS/FM patients. My colleague Tracey Beaulne, ND, who works clinically with Dr. Bested in Toronto, has seen numerous patients come to her with shopping bags filled with supplements as a result of self-prescriptions *and* visits to certain other NDs. As I mention in the supplement chapter, there are more than two hundred supplements touted as beneficial for CFS/FM, yet from my perspective only a handful may really help. I recommend you tell your ND that you prefer to keep the supplements to a bare minimum.

Second is the practice of techniques/modalities that are outside of the scope of naturopathic education. In an age when science is validating some of the health-promoting ideals of NDs, some continue to utilize dubious allergy tests, iridology, pseudoscientific measurements of oxidative stress, and other interventions that are not part of naturopathic education, and furthermore have been shown by modern research to be useless.

Some practitioners cannot let go of the disproved; instead, they ignore the promise of science. If you are a little skeptical of a gadget, machine, device, or intervention, ask about its validity and inquire about its publication in a reputable science journal. I would also recommend asking if training related to a questionable machine or intervention was conducted in the context of the ND degree program. Most often there is no science supporting these devices, and the outfits hawking them normally conduct the training. Keep in mind that questionable interventions can be a very lucrative business for practitioners and are most often nothing more than expensive placebos. If it seems too good to be true, it probably is.

States Currently Regulating Naturopathic Medicine		
Alaska	Kansas	Vermont
Arizona	Maine	Washington
California	Montana	U.S. territories:
Connecticut	New Hampshire	Puerto Rico and
District of Columbia	Oregon	Virgin Islands
Hawaii	Utah	

A legislative push is underway in New York. See www.nyanp.org.

CHIROPRACTIC

No medical profession can match the training and education in therapeutic spinal manipulation as is required of chiropractors. Four years of full-time graduate education, including the basic medical sciences and standardized national board exams have established chiropractic as a regulated profession with high standards. Chiropractic interventions involve the corrections of subluxations (misalignments) that interfere with normal physiology and vital energy flow. Chiropractors employ the "adjustment," technically referred to as spinal manipulative therapy, to correct subluxations and improve health. The preponderance of evidence from scientific studies shows that chiropractic is indeed beneficial in low back pain.

What about CFS/FM? There is little evidence that chiropractic is beneficial in CFS, though there is some evidence from one Canadian study that shows chiropractic may result in minor improvements in FM symptoms. The study, published in a chiropractic journal called the *Journal of Manipulative and Physiological Therapeutics*, showed significant improvements in range of motion and decreased self-reports of pain. However, there were no significant improvements in the defining and overall symptoms of FM. Still, survey-based research shows that between 20 and 50 percent of FM patients seek chiropractic care and of those patients about half report some symptom relief. Those are not bad numbers and indicate that chiropractic may be a suitable complement to standard care in FM.

Chiropractors and NDs are trained in the use of legitimate machines called interferential electrotherapy and therapeutic ultrasound. These devices may be of real value in FM, according to exciting new research published in 2003. Individually, both machines have been shown to be beneficial in musculoskeletal pain conditions by various mechanisms, but most notably through improving blood flow, stimulating voluntary muscles, and having a positive effect on cellular membrane permeability.

The study, published in the prestigious journal *Pain*, showed that combining interferential electrotherapy and therapeutic ultrasound could not only reduce overall body pain and pain at the tender points, but could also improve sleep quality and decrease morning fatigue. What is so impressive about this study is that it was controlled through the use of a sham group where patients had the same treatment but without the actual electric current or ultrasound turned on. The results were statistically higher in the active treatment group. Improving sleep quality is so important in CFS/FM, and these results suggest, at least in FM, that it may be worth asking your chiropractor to combine these therapies along with correction of subluxations.

Risks/Caveats
The risk of chiropractic is often overstated in the media and on some Web sites. Serious adverse events are reported to be only 0.0001 percent of all treatments. Some CFS/FM patients report mild aggravations of symptoms after chiropractic treatments, particularly adjustments without adequate soft tissue massage and stretching.

A serious concern is that a growing number of chiropractors hold themselves out to be alternative medicine "experts" without the appropriate education. Keep in mind that less than 10 percent of chiropractic education is outside of the neuromuscularskeletal system; there is rarely formal training in botanical medicine and homeopathy and only relatively few hours spent in basic/clinical nutrition. In addition, there are no specific licensing board exams where these alternative modalities are examined for competency within chiropractic. If you are looking for advice *outside* of traditional spinal manipulation and electrotherapy, see a chiropractor who has made the educational commitment to obtain advanced training in complementary therapies and nutrition. There are a growing number of chiropractors with advanced training in nutrition or with ND credentials. Outside of that, there are plenty of chiropractors now working with NDs to ensure that a more comprehensive approach is available to patients.

MASSAGE THERAPY

Manual manipulation of soft tissue for therapeutic purposes is one of the oldest forms of treatment. There are countless forms of massage therapy, with a variety of techniques used in clinical practice. Two forms of massage have emerged as the most popular in North America: Swedish massage and shiatsu.

Swedish massage, as practiced today, involves muscle manipulation, including light sweeping strokes to deeper, more vigorous rubbing, kneading, and compression. Swedish massage moves lymph and blood through your tissue and helps remove lactic acid from the muscles. Shiatsu is an ancient healing art, originating in China and developed further in Japan. Shiatsu is a complement to acupuncture, as it involves the application of pressure along energy meridians, the same twelve elemental meridians used in acupuncture. Shiatsu practitioners may apply pressure and stretching with their thumbs, knuckles, palms, and even elbows to move trapped qi (vital energy in the meridians, pronounced *chee*). The improper flow of qi is thought to be the cause of chronic pain and fatigue.

There is no question that massage therapy, whatever the form, can result in significant physiological changes in the body, particularly the dampening of the sympathetic nervous system. Massage therapy can induce a great sense of relaxation, reduce muscle tension, increase digestion, and reduce overall stress.

While there are effects mediated by direct mechanical pressure, perhaps it is the human touch that conveys the greatest benefits of massage. A five-week study involving CFS patients shows just how important the human touch can be. Patients had a proper, hands-on massage or a massage with a rolling device that was not turned on. The hands-on massage led to greater improvements in depressive and bodily symptoms in CFS. There is also some research indicating that massage therapy may be valuable in FM, at least in the short-term. Research on massage therapy within other conditions has shown it to increase natural killer cell activity (this would be of benefit in CFS), lift mood, reduce stress hormone release, and increase levels of certain mood-regulating neurotransmitters. The results of these studies are very encouraging and support massage's role in true, holistic care.

There are some other, less well-known techniques that are utilized by massage therapists, including reflexology and cranio-sacral massage. Reflexology is massage based around a system of points in the hands and feet thought to correspond, or "reflex," to all areas of the body. Cranio-sacral technique involves subtle readjustments thought to influence rhythmic pulsations of spinal fluid. There is no scientific evidence that cranio-sacral technique is of value, and the ideas behind it actually challenge known concepts of anatomy. However, there are plenty of anecdotal reports of benefit, and many CFS/FM patients find it helpful. Reflexology, on the other hand, has had some favorable controlled studies in support of it. In the journal *Multiple Sclerosis*, patients with multiple sclerosis were randomized to received either actual reflexology or a sham massage. After eleven weeks, the reflexology group had significant improvements in various motor and sensory outcomes. Previous controlled research has shown that reflexology may be of benefit in premenstrual syndrome. Not every study of reflexology has been positive, but it is an area that warrants further investigation.

What about the practitioners: are there standards of education and qualifying requirements? The answer, within a growing number of states and provinces, is yes. More than half of states require that someone who calls him- or herself a massage therapist be duly licensed to do so. Licensure (or registration in Canada) allows the practitioners to call themselves LMT/RMT, licensed/registered massage therapist, and this designation is not easily obtained. It requires a tremendous amount of hard work and the passage of difficult board exams that cover the basic medical sciences; some states also require practical and oral exams. Generally, at least five hundred hours of classroom and clinical coursework are required before a candidate can sit for board exams in the United States; in Canada, it's more than two thousand hours! To be honest, there is an under-appreciation of the work necessary to become a LMT or RMT. Licensure is determined on a state and provincial level, so I would recommend contacting the following organizations for further information; they represent only qualified LMTs in the United States (American Massage Therapy Association, www.amtamassage.org) and RMTs in Canada (Canadian Massage Therapist Alliance, www.cmta.ca). Massage should be considered a valuable complement to standard care. Licensed practitioners are highly trained and knowledgable.

Risks/Caveats
There are few medical interventions as safe as massage therapy; the most recent published review reports that serious adverse events are rarities. Many CFS/FM patients have tried massage therapy, and the majority report it to be beneficial. A few patients I interviewed stated that more vigorous, deep-tissue massage made pain and fatigue worse. This shouldn't be cause to abandon massage therapy completely; instead, talk to your massage therapist—an LMT or RMT will adapt any massage technique to your comfort level. Massage therapy, like other forms of complementary care, is not a substitute for appropriate medical care.

ACUPUNCTURE

Now practiced throughout the world, acupuncture originated in China and makes up one part of what is known as traditional Asian medicine (TAM). Asian herbal medicine is the other main TAM component, and the two are probably best used together. Acupuncture involves insertion of a needle into the skin, making contact with underlying tissue in specific points along twelve meridians or energy channels. It is through the meridians that qi, the vital energy responsible for nourishing and defending the body, is said to flow. A disturbance or blockage of qi can lead to chronic fatigue and chronic pain. Needling (or pressing in acupressure) of points is intended to gain access to the meridians in an effort to restore energy flow and promote healing.

A number of investigators have attempted to substantiate the presence of meridians and points or at least determine how different they may be from surrounding tissue. Perhaps the most exciting of these efforts is that by Dr. Helene Langevin and colleagues from the University of Vermont. They have found that there is an overlap between acupuncture points and sites where connective tissue are joined. Explanations for the physiological effects of needling in the meeting points of these sheets of tissue have been given, and hopefully further research will uncover more of the scientific anatomy and physiology of the meridians. It has been shown in studies over the years that acupuncture can stimulate the release of pain-modulating opioids and mood-regulating neurotransmitters such as serotonin.

Research indicates that acupuncture can be of real value in FM, particularly in pain management, sleep, and depressive symptoms. Some of the better-controlled studies with FM patients have used legitimate acupuncture and "sham" acupuncture (i.e., needling off the meridians) as a control. Acupuncture treatment has also been shown to increase blood flow and temperature at the tender points in FM patients. There are enough controlled acupuncture studies to justify giving it a try if you have FM or pain in CFS. The evidence for acupuncture is limited in CFS, although research published in the *Journal of Chinese Medicine* indicates that it may be helpful with some of the symptoms, including fatigue.

Once again, regulation of acupuncture is controlled at the state and provincial level; for more information and to find a properly trained and qualified professional, contact the National Certification Commission of Acupuncture and Oriental Medicine (NCCAOM) in the United States (www.nccaom.org);

in Canada, contact the Chinese Medicine and Acupuncture Association of Canada (www.cmaac.ca).

Risks/Caveats

The risk of adverse events is reported to be very low when treated by a properly trained acupuncturist. CFS/FM patients may be sensitive to the fumes of moxa, an herbal stick that is sometimes used to warm the needles. Be aware that not every licensed acupuncturist is the ideal candidate for initiating CFS/FM treatment. CFS/FM are complex conditions and can be made worse by well-meaning practitioners. Sadly, there are too many "cookbook" acupuncturists in North America who rely on a few well-known pain or energy modulating points. In the *Journal of Chinese Medicine*, Giovanni Maciocia (arguably the most knowledgeable acupuncturist in the West) describes how complex CFS is and how delicate the treatment needs to be. Certain basic points may be helpful in alleviating pain in FM, but for both CFS and FM, a proper work-up should explore the diagnoses from a traditional Asian (TAM) perspective.

HOMEOPATHY

Possibly the most frequently used form of CAM, homeopathy remains steeped in controversy. The word *homeopathy* translates from Greek as "similar disease." This means that if you give a homeopathic substance (ultra-dilute plant, mineral, or animal extract) to a healthy subject, they will display symptoms that are similar to those individuals who are actually experiencing a disease/condition. By contrast, that same homeopathic substance should lead to an improvement in those who actually have the disease or condition. Let's take the homeopathic remedy Rhus tox, well-known as an arthritis remedy, and shown in one controlled study published in the *British Medical Journal* to be of value in FM. Giving Rhus tox (derived from the poison ivy plant) to a person with arthritis or FM may improve symptoms, while giving it to a healthy person may lead to arthritic or FM symptoms. This is called the principle of similars, or like cures like.

Clearly, this idea is bound to cause controversy, but where homeopathy really moves away from traditional thinking is in the assumption that the more diluted a remedy is, the stronger it becomes. A standard potency of homeopathic remedies in health food stores is usually called a 6C. What this means is that the remedy, let's say Rhus tox, has been diluted in this fashion: 1 part of the botanical Rhus tox tincture is diluted into 99 parts water/alcohol, then 1 part of this new diluted mix is added to 99 parts water until the process has been done six times over (diluted 1:100 six times). This particular dilution is considered one of the weaker remedies. By the time the most potent remedies are prepared, they may not even contain a single molecule of the original substance. While there really is no proven scientific justification for a biological effect, some physicists use "quantum physics" to explain the effects. Quantum physics explains invisible units of energy that are known as quanta. They have proposed that electromagnetic energy in the medicines may interact with the body.

So, homeopathy hasn't been fully explained at the present time, but the real question is, What is the clinical evidence? There is enough evidence from controlled trials to at least support keeping an open mind, according to a recent critical review of homeopathy published in the *Annals of Internal Medicine*. Three large reviews of placebo-controlled trials indicate that homeopathy is more effective than placebo, while one concluded that it was similar to placebo. A large number of the clinical studies to date have been of poor quality, but it is interesting to note that the better quality studies in recent years have been favorable toward homeopathy in the treatment of allergies, asthma, and childhood diarrhea. A separate study published in the *International Journal of Alternative and Complementary Medicine* showed that appropriately prescribed remedies were more beneficial than placebo in CFS.

One of the main problems with the single-remedy controlled trials in homeopathy is that using one remedy in a study of forty to fifty patients (versus placebo) goes against the practice of classical homeopathy—a single remedy would never be prescribed for an entire patient population. Individual differences, even subtle ones, will alter the remedy chosen. If one hundred FM patients showed up in the office of a classical homeopath, very few would probably end up with, for example, Rhus tox. Some practitioners of homeopathy use a blend of different remedies in one prescription; this is called clinical homeopathy, and despite being more of a shotgun technique, it can be equally complex.

Either way, a good homeopath, or physician practicing homeopathy, will consider your entire person, including your constellation of CFS/FM symptoms and life experiences, before making a remedy choice. Homeopathic case taking is an art, one that is time-consuming and extremely detailed. Practitioners who appear to get the best clinical results are individuals who can capture subtleties and make an appropriate match to the remedy based on knowledge of the 2,500 homeopathic substances. The evidence to date suggests that, even in the absence of a known method of action, homeopathy warrants further investigation and may be a worthwhile consideration in FM.

Risks/Caveats

Homeopathy is not associated with significant adverse events. It is reported that about 20 percent of patients taking homeopathic remedies have an aggravation of symptoms, a so-called "healing crisis" that represents the road to recovery. Healing is said to progress from the deepest part of the body to the extremities, from the emotional and mental aspects to the physical, and from the upper part of the body to the lower parts of the body. Due to possible worsening of symptoms, CFS/FM patients should be cautious with self-prescribing homeopathic remedies. If you would like to give homeopathy a try, look for someone with experience. Many homeopathic providers in North America are not medically trained; look for MDs, DOs, and dentists who are members of the American Institute of Homeopathy (www.homeopathyusa.org) or an ND, particularly one who is a Diplomate of the Homeopathic Academy of Naturopathic Physicians (www.hanp.net). The most serious risk of homeopathic medicine is when it is substituted for appropriate medical care.

Aromatherapy

Probably the most under-valued CAM modality, aromatherapy is emerging as a science-based discipline. The medicinal use of plant essential oils can be traced back to ancient China and the Indian subcontinent. Until recently, most of the evidence pertaining to essential oils was based on anecdotal case reports. Thanks to some incredible, well-designed studies, we have learned that odors can have a profound effect on cognition and emotion. The mere discussion of an aroma can lead to numerous associated memories, which in turn are attached to emotions. The influence of scent over emotions is a result of an intricate neurological connection between the olfactory nerves (smell) and the limbic system (emotional centers).

It is well known that when olfactory nerves are damaged in animals, symptoms resembling depression and anxiety often result. It is also interesting to note that there is a high concentration of omega-3 fatty acids (docosahexaenoic acid, DHA) within the olfactory nerves of animals and that deficiencies of omega-3 fatty acids cause a marked reduction in DHA within the olfactory bulb. Depressed patients are known to have diminished smell sensitivity, and when in remission, they, and patients with seasonal affective disorder (SAD), have been shown to have an increased acuity for smells versus healthy subjects. Omega-3 fatty acid deficiencies that have been consistently observed in depression may be playing a role in altered smell sensitivity. This is an exciting area of research, and hopefully further investigations will explore this connection.

In the meantime, the effects of both pleasant and unpleasant odors have been shown to have physiological effects on the human nervous system. In an interesting study published in 2003, Dr. Naohiko Inoue and colleagues from Kyoto University in Japan showed that high-intensity jasmine odor could increase parasympathetic nervous system activity in those who liked the smell and increase sympathetic nervous system activity (increased stress) among those who did not like the smell. This seems reasonable, but what was really interesting was that at very low levels, jasmine had a positive influence on the parasympathetic nervous system in all subjects, even those claiming not to like jasmine aroma.

A U.S. study, presented at the 2002 annual meeting of the Society for Psychophysiological Research, showed that a faint odor of jasmine infused in sleeping quarters resulted in less tossing and turning, and subjects were less anxious upon waking. The investigators had participants sleep in rooms for three nights; each night they were infused with either jasmine, lavender, or no scent. Subjectively, those sleepers in the jasmine room felt more alert later in the day, particularly during the afternoon hours. From a scientific perspective there were also some key objective findings. When participants were asked to match numbers to symbols the following day, sleeping in the jasmine-infused room led to higher scores of mental function. In the same study, lavender was also helpful, but not to the same degree as jasmine. In an interesting correlate with the Japanese study, many of the sleepers were unaware of the scent at all because the infusion amounts were tiny, yet the aroma appeared to have physiological and psychological effects.

In another important study, Dr. Mark Moss and colleagues from the University of Northumbria's (UK) Human Cognitive Neuroscience Unit showed that essential oils of lavender and rosemary have quite different effects on human cognition. The study, involving 140 healthy adults, revealed that those exposed to lavender had a significant decrease in working memory as well as a decrease in the reaction times for both memory- and attention-based tasks. On the contrary, rosemary produced a significant enhancement of performance related to memory. Following the battery of performance tests, the lavender and control (no scent) groups were significantly less alert than the rosemary group. As for mood, both the lavender and rosemary groups were more content than the control group. Lavender appears to be a sedating aroma; previous studies have shown that it can improve mood and prolong physiological markers of relaxation when added to a footbath. The study by Dr. Moss and colleagues was recently published in the *International Journal of Neuroscience*, and hopefully it is the beginning of a new wave of scientific evaluations of aromatherapy.

A series of case studies using aromatherapy in FM has been published and indicates that there may be some short-term benefits, including reductions in pain and enhanced sleep. Based on this research, an experienced Finnish aromatherapist, Ulla-Maija Grace, has brought Fibromix to the market. "Fibromix" is a specific blend of essential oils reported to be of value in FM. It is available through a Finland-based company called Aromatica (e-mail: info@aromatica.fi). The value of the aromatherapy used in the FM patients dissipates over time as patients begin to find a scent "unwanted," and it should be pointed out that the case studies are far from a proper controlled trial. Still, aromatherapy may be worth trying for occasional use, mainly as a form of relaxation and perhaps as a means to diminish some of the symptoms.

Risks/Caveats

Despite chemical sensitivities, most CFS/FM patients I interviewed indicate that they tolerate low doses of essential oils quite well. Problems may arise when the oils are synthetic or chemically altered. Essential oils should not be taken internally or used undiluted on the skin.

Aromatherapy is an unregulated CAM modality; professional standards are lacking, and despite the advances in science, exaggerated claims of the benefits of aromatherapy abound. Most practitioners of aromatherapy are not medically trained, and although it may be an excellent complement to standard care, it should never be considered a substitute.

CONCLUSIONS

CAM therapies continue to be a topic of fierce debate, with proponents and opponents digging in their heels in a standoff that will ultimately be decided by science. Of course some individuals, both practitioners and patients alike, will hold fast to their beliefs, even when science has disproved a remedy, device, or technique. On the other hand, so-called CFS and FM expert physicians (with very little/no CAM experience) are often quick to slam the door on potentially valuable CAM modalities as a means to help reduce some symptoms and improve quality of life. These individuals have already made up their minds, and it's a sad, one-dimensional view.

For this reason, CFS/FM patients need to be well-educated not only about their illness but also about the providers who become involved. Any patient with a chronic illness is particularly vulnerable to the excesses of CAM, particularly its exorbitant claims and false promises.

CAM becomes a real concern when:

1. It is used as an alternative/substitute for appropriate diagnosis and medical care.
2. It uses costly diagnostic techniques and treatments that have been shown to be useless.
3. It involves the prescription of inordinate amounts of supplements and botanicals.
4. Providers make promises they can't deliver on.

The CAM modalities discussed in this chapter are generally safe; the effectiveness of some appears to be legitimate and of some value to CFS/FM patients when used in the context of appropriate medical care. CAM practioners provide a precious commodity that has slipped away from orthodox medicine—

time. The clinician-patient bond that develops as result of adequate time and interacting with the patient is akin to the placebo response and can have a tremendous influence on healing.

CFS/FM patients may want to explore the CAM avenues discussed above. Remember, it is important to inform your MD or DO if you are seeing a CAM provider.

CHAPTER SUMMARY

- Complementary and alternative medicine (CAM) modalities include naturopathic medicine, chiropractic, massage therapy, acupuncture, homeopathy, and aromatherapy.
- CAM modalities are frequently used by CFS/FM patients and generally are reported to be a valuable adjunct.
- Unlike most mainstream physicians, CAM practitioners generally have the luxury of time, which, in turn, may be interpreted as extended care.
- CFS/FM patients should always disclose CAM use to the treating physicians. Patients cannot control the response of the provider, it may be supportive or judgmental, but in any case, the use of CAM is your right.
- There may be treatment value to CAM modalities, but there are also associated risks, which range from a worsening of CFS/FM to a lightening of your purse.
- CAM is never a substitute for appropriate medical intervention.

HERMAN®

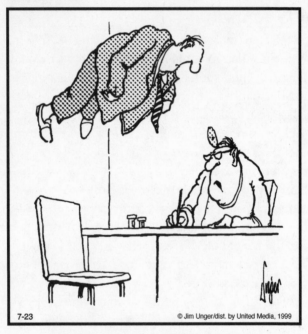

"I'll give you something for gas."

CHAPTER EIGHT

PHARMACEUTICAL TREATMENTS

In my practice we try nonprescription methods to treat symptoms first because I work with a naturopathic doctor. If the symptoms are treated early on by the other modalities, prescription medications may not be necessary. Often, however, by the time I see the patients, symptomatic treatment with pharmaceutical drugs is necessary due to the severity of the symptoms. Patients with multiple chemical sensitivity may not be able to tolerate many of the medications as a result of their reactions to chemicals and medications. Sometimes patients even have "paradoxical reactions," meaning that the medication has the opposite reaction to what was intended. For example, a patient given an anti-anxiety medication might suffer a panic attack after taking the medication. This is not common, but it does happen with very chemically sensitive patients. I cannot stress enough the importance of learning as many tools to cope with your illness as possible, including relaxation techniques, meditation, visualization, sleep hygiene, gradual mobilization, massage, aromatherapy, exercise, pacing, etc. Medication should be used as an additional tool to recovery, but not the only tool. Medications are often used for symptomatic relief of sleep difficulties, pain, depression, and treatable infections. This section is intended only as a guideline; each patient must be individually assessed and reassessed on a regular basis by their doctor for their particular problems and treatments.

MEDICATIONS USED TO TREAT CFS/FM

There are no interventions or medications that are universally effective in treating the symptoms of all CFS/FM patients—some medications may be helpful for most, but none for all. The challenge for treating physicians is that many patients with CFS/FM cannot tolerate medications in the usual starting doses. Instead, the medication must be started at lower doses (often one-quarter of the usual dose) and gradually built up. Just like with exercising, the rule for CFS/FM patients is *start low and go slow*. Doctors must use a trial-and-error method in choosing medications and dosages that will help to make you feel better but at the same time not aggravate your symptoms. This chapter discusses some of the more commonly prescribed medications used to treat the symptoms of CFS/FM. Just to stress again, there is no magic pill for any of the symptoms in CFS/FM. There must be a lot of hard work by yourself and your doctor, trying various medications to see which one or combinations work best in your particular body. It really helps when you keep a diary of your symptoms and their intensity so that you can take it to your doctor's visits. This will help you and your doctor determine which medication is working best.

One of the best things about the human body is our ability to forget a symptom when it disappears. Kind of like forgetting the severe pain of childbirth—which allows you to consider having a second child. If a woman actually remembered the pain of child birth on an ongoing basis, most families would only have one child.

Often patients forget to tell me about the symptoms that disappear, an indication that a medication is working. That's why keeping activity logs and tracking not only problems but also improvements is so important.

SLEEP MEDICATION

By the time patients see me they have usually already experienced ongoing sleep disorders, sometimes for years. Since I am a "doctor of last resort," this is often where I begin to try to help patients. After I have gone through the sleep hygiene routine and the other modalities to help sleep have been exhausted, I explore the use of medications to help a patient sleep. Just to be clear, there is not a pill out there that will bring back your restorative deep sleep, the problem that all CFS/FM patients have. The sleeping pills are used in order to help you feel that you have given your brain a break for at least a few hours. The pills will not therefore make you feel refreshed in the morning; some pills will even make you feel groggier in the morning. This is the art of medicine—trying to find a medication that will help you feel you have had some sleep without leaving you feeling hungover in the morning. Each patient is different, requiring different medication and different doses.

At the top of the activity log (see page 54) is a place for you to record the quality of your sleep and the number of hours that you sleep each night. This is a good way to help you and your doctor figure out if a new medication is working. If you do not write things down odds are you will forget, since loss of short-term memory is part of the illness.

Some of the medications listed here are not considered sleeping medication or hypnotics. Muscle relaxants, antidepressants, pain medications, and anticonvulsants can help to improve sleep quality as well. When doctors use medications in these ways, they are using them in an "off-label" way. In other words, they are using them for their side effects and not their originally intended use. This is one of the ways that the practice of medicine evolves. The nice thing is that when more than one symptom is present as is the case in CFS/FM, you get a better bang for your buck.

The medications listed below have been found to be beneficial in improving sleep quality in CFS/FM. Some are prescription while others are over-the-counter medications. They are from different categories of drugs. They include medication to treat nausea, depression, muscle spasms, anxiety, and insomnia. A list like this emphasizes again that one size does not fit all. Two drug names are given in the list—the first is the chemical name or the generic name and the second is the trade name or the manufacturer's name. The list is by no means all-inclusive, but these are some of the medications I've found can help patients sleep. Another thing I have observed is that in some patients more than one medication may be needed to induce sleep and to keep patients asleep throughout the night. Treatment is very individualized and has to take into account the entire drug complex the patient is taking. Some drugs are not compatible with certain types of antidepressants. For this reason, always get all of your prescription drugs from one pharmacist and *always* check to be sure that a new medication is compatible with the other pharmaceutical medications and herbal medications you take before you start taking it. Pharmacists have access to online computer drug compatibility data that many doctors do not have in their offices.

The doses listed here are the typical starting doses listed for non-CFS/FM patients, so one quarter of the listed dose may in fact be enough for some patients who are very sensitive to the effects of medications. For more details about medications please refer to the *Journal of Chronic Fatigue Syndrome*, Volume 11, Number 1, 2003.

Pharmaceuticals for Sleep Disturbance
Dimenhydrinate/Gravol 25–50 mg
Tryptophan/Tryptan 500mg–3 gm
Zopiclone/Imovane 5–15 mg
Clonazepam/Rivotril 0.5–2 mg
Doxepin/Sinequan 2–200 mg
Amitriptyline/Elavil 5–50 mg
Trazodone/Desyrel 50–150 mg
Cyclobenzaprine/Flexeril 10 mg
Mirtazapine/Remeron 15–30 mg
Bromazepam/Lectopam 1–3 mg
Zolpidem/Ambien 5–10 mg (available only in the United States)

Patients often say to me that they don't want to take a pill because they fear they will become "addicted" to the medication. In the case of CFS/FM, you have a *documented* sleep disorder. You are taking the medication in order to improve your sleep so that you can function better and have a better quality of life. My suggestion is that if your sleep improves on the medication, then take it. I find that when you feel that you have a better night's sleep you start to improve physically. And often, if you don't sleep, you don't heal. What I mean by having a better night's sleep is that you don't spend the entire night tossing and turning and looking at the clock to see what time it is. You feel as if you have had some sleep. Would you tell a diabetic not to take his insulin? Of course not. Why? Because he needs it. If you have a sleep disorder and you have had a sleep study done that shows lack of deep sleep and multiple interruptions during your sleep, you will probably benefit from some type of medication to help you with your sleep on an ongoing basis.

Safety Issue

If you have been on any of the medications in this chapter for a while, your body is used to them. This is called tolerance. Your body will have a physical tolerance to the medication, so that if you decide to stop the medication you will need to taper off the medication slowly with your doctor's supervision. If you stop suddenly, you will have expected medication withdrawal symptoms—for example, with sleep medication, you will not sleep the whole night. This is extremely anxiety producing and may cause a panic attack in some cases, so avoid this if at all possible. However, there can be other severe uncomfortable side effects, depending on the particular medication being stopped. Each medication is different, so again check with your doctor before you change or discontinue any prescribed medication.

Because of the dangers of withdrawal symptoms and drug interactions, I recommend that you carry a card in your wallet that lists all of your medications in case you are in an accident and you cannot speak. The doctors in the emergency room need to know that you have been on a long-term sleeping medication or an antidepressant or pain medication so that they can continue the medication in the hospital—or a medication similar to it—to prevent you from accidentally experiencing medication withdrawal.

HYPNOTICS (e.g., Zopiclone/Imovane, Zolpidem/Ambien)

There are many sleep-inducing medications available. Hypnotics are interesting because they may increase the amount of Stage III and IV deep sleep. They work well in many patients alone or in combination with Tryptophan. The doses are very individualized. In the United States patients report that Ambien is often helpful.

BENZODIAZEPINES (e.g., clonazepam)

Although fatigue is a major symptom of CFS (and can be found in FM too), patients often report feeling "wound up" or "tired yet wired." If you are wired, relaxation techniques can help your medications work more effectively. Benzodiazepines are known as sedative-hypnotics. They can help to calm you, reduce anxiety, and treat insomnia. They work by depressing a part of the brain called the reticular activating system that regulates how active the brain is. They also help with restless leg syndrome if this is a part of the sleep disturbance. Clonazepam often works well by itself or in combination with Sinequan.

PAIN MEDICATION

Pain medication includes anything that you put into your body to combat pain. It includes over-the-counter medications and herbs such as aspirin, Tylenol, Advil, and Lakota. Often patients forget to mention the fact that they are taking over-the-counter pills and herbs in addition to their prescribed medications. It is vital to tell your doctor everything. Why? Because all of these things are, biochemically, medicine at a cellular level and have the potential to interact with one another and magnify the effect in the body. Pharmacists have access to drug and herbal interaction charts. Your doctor can phone for information if he/she doesn't have on-line access in his/her medical office. The total load of over-the-counter medications, prescription medications, and herbal medications all must be detoxified by the liver and kidneys before they leave the body. So work together with your doctors, both medical and naturopathic, so they know the entire picture and not just a piece of the medicinal puzzle.

Omega-3 and -6 Oils

The more the omega oils are studied, the more it is realized that these need to be in balance to support healing in the body. This is particularly true in the area of pain management. Supplementing with these oils in a balanced ratio helps reduce the inflammatory process by reducing the amount of inflammatory cytokines in the body. In the CFS/FM patient population, this is extremely important. In fact, some of my patients have been able to reduce the amount of pain medication required when they use the proper supplements and vitamins and rid their diets of additives, pesticides, and food allergies. Please see chapters 4 and 5 for more information.

NON-STEROIDAL ANTI-INFLAMMATORY DRUGS (NSAIDS, e.g., Ibuprofen, Naproxen)

Medications in the anti-inflammatory group work much better if the previous corrections have been made in the different areas of the body: eliminating sugars, pesticides, and food allergies; balancing the omega-3 and -6 oils; exercising or walking as tolerated; practicing relaxation techniques and massage; and using a sleep routine. All of these changes will help the body reduce inflammation at the cellular level so less medication is needed. The drugs included as anti-inflammatories start with the common over-the-counter drugs aspirin and ibuprofen. They work by inhibiting the production of prostaglandins, hormone-like substances that cause swelling and pain (inflammation) in the injured tissue. By blocking the production of prostaglandins in the tissue, stimulation of the nerve endings is prevented so that no pain signal passes to the brain. CFS/FM patients commonly use NSAIDs to reduce inflammation, and some report them to be quite helpful while others find no benefit. NSAIDs have been shown to be effective in the treatment of the following overlapping conditions common to CFS/FM patients: osteoarthritis, rheumatoid arthritis, and chronic low back pain.

Some prostaglandins are beneficial and are involved in maintaining the protective fluid lining in the stomach. Therefore, one of the major side effects of NSAIDs is the risk of developing stomach upset, stomach ulcers, and blood in the stool. COX-2 inhibitors are a newer class of NSAIDs. Unfortunately, COX-2 inhibitors have been associated with side effects including heart problems and stroke. As a result, they have been either withdrawn completely or used much more cautiously than when they were initially introducted. In my opinion, medication from this group is best used in a pulse fashion, meaning they can often be used successfully intermittently or for short periods of time in the patient who has been properly screened for safe use.

Muscle Relaxants (e.g., Flexeril, Baclofen)

Research supports the use of the muscle relaxant cyclobenzaprine in the treatment of CFS/FM patients with pain, sleep disorders, or irritable bowel syndrome. FM sufferers seem to have less pain and fatigue, fewer painful trigger points, and improved sleep on this drug. Tizanidine (Zanaflex) is another muscle relaxant that has shown to be useful in the treatment of the following conditions associated with CFS/FM: chronic daily headaches, low back pain, sleep, and pain. It is reported that Tizanidine can reduce the amount of substance P, an important consideration in patients with FM. Substance P is the neurotransmitter involved in the pain response. If you bite into a hot chili pepper, substance P will be released and, well, you know the consequences. FM patients have been shown to have abnormally high levels of substance P, much higher than healthy adults and CFS patients. Diazepam/ Valium is an excellent muscle relaxant that can be used. It is best used intermittently for pulsed periods due to the loss of effectiveness over time and the possibility of tolerance when severe muscle spasm is present.

Drugs for Pain (Analgesics)

Analgesics relieve pain. They include common over-the-counter drugs such as acetaminophen (better known as Tylenol) and stronger narcotic prescription drugs including codeine, oxycodone, tramadol hydrochloride, morphine, and fentanyl. Like NSAIDs, acetaminophen only provides minor pain relief. Stronger pain relief may be achieved when acetaminophen is combined with codeine, as in Tylenol #3 or Percoset (Tylenol combined with oxycodone). Narcotics are available by prescription only.

An adequate trial of non-opiod analgesics should be carried out before narcotics are used. Most patients do not want to initiate narcotic treatment and would prefer to try to live with pain levels of 8 to 10 out of 10; such is the fear of addiction. Addiction is defined by the 4Cs: cravings, control, consumption, and consequences. This means that when a patient is addicted they constantly crave the drug; they lose control while using the drug or get high; they keep increasing their consumption of the drug even when increasing the dose has no effect and they risk losing their jobs, families, etc.; and they take it without regard for the consequences of taking the drug. The risk of addiction, however, is low when dealing with organic pain, as in CFS/FM patients who have been properly screened for a history of past recreational drug and alcohol abuse. To date, addiction has not been a problem in my patients who are on pain medication for chronic pain. I checked with the expert pain specialist in my area who lectures about chronic non-malignant pain, Dr. Roman Jovey, and this has also been his experience.

The treatment of chronic, non-malignant pain is newly recognized in medicine. The treatment of cancer (malignant) pain is a better understood area. Many doctors have not been formally trained to use narcotics in the treatment of CFS/FM. Therefore, if you have severe pain you may need to be referred to a pain specialist for assessment and initial treatment. Under guidance of the specialist, your general practitioner may then continue with therapy if your doctor has these prescribing privileges. The purpose of medications is not to completely eliminate pain; rather it is to make it more manageable and improve the patient's quality of life. So, for example, a patient who has a pain level of 10 out of 10, which is the most severe pain, would hope to bring the pain down to a more manageable level at about 5 out of 10 with the use of medication. Using pain medication also demands personal responsibility from the patient. Sometimes patients are asked to enter into a contract with the doctor when prescription pain medications are used. This includes full disclosure of all pain medications and treatments, past drug and alcohol history, family drug and alcohol history, agreement for only one physician to prescribe pain medication, keeping a pain diary to record pain levels and the amount and time the medication was taken, and agreeing to random drug testing. This information is available online in a publication by the College of Physicians and Surgeons of Ontario. (For the *Reference Guide for Clinicians on Evidence-Based Recommendations for Medical Management of Chronic Non-Malignant Pain*, please see www.cpso.on.ca/publication; scroll down to page 19.) This is where I practice medicine and I am governed by this college. Each state or province has guidelines that determine how physicians can practice medicine. Find out what the regulations are for your area.

Doctors are required to keep records of all narcotic medications and to document the effects of the pain medication in use. For better pain control and to eliminate peaks and valleys of pain control it is advantageous to the patient to switch from short-acting to long-acting analgesics if possible. Long-acting narcotics usually have *contin* as part of their name. The contins are usually better for the patient as there are fewer side effects. For example, hydromorph contin/hydromorphone, the longer-acting slow-release form of morphine, has fewer side effects than morphine, which is the shorter-acting form. The longer-acting or contin products last for six to twelve hours depending on the individual medication. In addition there are long-acting patches such as the fentanyl patch Duragesic. It lasts for approximately three days in most patients. Longer-acting medications give better pain control to the patient and as a result patients have a better quality of life. Usually when you are on long-term pain management you are required to visit your doctor on a regular basis, monthly or even more often. Medication is often given out at best on a monthly basis and at worst on a daily basis by the pharmacist. If you are taking a long-term pain medication, you must not stop it on your own. Sudden cessation of the medication will cause symptoms of withdrawal, because your body does have a physical tolerance to the medication when you are taking it. Not all medications work in each patient. Research has shown that our body has at least four different pain receptors in the brain. Certain drugs probably work better with different receptors. Who knows—in the future, before beginning pain medication, doctors may order a blood test to find out which pain receptors you have in your brain so that he or she can predict which type of pain medication will work best in your body. With the availability of the human genetic code, "Star Trek" medicine is just around the corner. As a medical doctor I am amazed at the huge number of research breakthroughs that occur almost weekly.

Pain medication of various kinds can be given by many different routes, including the following: pills by mouth (e.g., Advil, morphine), patches on the skin (e.g., Duragesic patch), cream on the skin (e.g., Voltaren anti-inflammatory cream), suppositories in the rectum (e.g., anti-nausea Stemetil), injections into the tender points (e.g., local anesthetic Xylocaine), or nerve blocks. Botox injections have also been successfully used if severe ongoing migraine headaches are a feature of fibromyalgia pain.

Any medication has potential side effects. Sometimes it is the side effect that determines which type of medication is more beneficial to the patient. You will discuss ahead of time the potential side effects with your doctor so that you will be aware of them and know how to handle them if they do happen to you. One of the most common side effects of narcotic pain medication is constipation. If the constipation is not managed, you will not be able to manage the pain medication. So odds are you will need to increase your fiber and possibly use medication such as a stool softener or laxative if you begin a narcotic medication. Another common side effect is initial drowsiness when the medication is started. For this reason it is always beneficial to start a new medication at night if possible. Until the dose is adjusted properly your doctor will ask that you not drive your car. When the medication has been properly adjusted it should not cause excessive drowsiness. Just because you are taking narcotic medication does not mean that you cannot function. In fact with less pain you ideally should have less fatigue and be able to do more over time. That is the purpose of the pain medication, to allow you to have a better quality of life.

Your doctor may not feel comfortable treating you with narcotic pain medication if you have had a history of drug or alcohol abuse because of the risk of addiction. If the doctor is not comfortable with your history of past addiction to drugs or alcohol, the doctor is not obliged to treat your pain with medication. He or she can try other non-medication modalities such as biofeedback or relaxation therapy or refer you to a pain specialist that has experience with chronic pain and addiction. These expert pain doctors are trained in the use of methadone at pain clinics that specialize in pain addiction and pain control in the addicted patients. This is a very complicated area of medicine and very few doctors are experienced enough to be able to deal with complicated cases of chronic pain and addiction. Usually these expert pain doctors are located in specially designated pain clinics.

If you are taking pain medication on a regular basis you will need to keep a pain diary with the level of pain on a scale of 1 to 10, your medications, time of medication, activities of daily living, and side effects of the medications. Your doctor will also keep track of these things on your chart, as shown below.

The 5 "A"s in the Patient's Chart on Pain Medication Documents

Analgesia, scale of 1 to 10

Activities of daily living (physical & psychosocial functioning)

Adverse effects

Aberrant drug-taking behaviors

Accurate medication recording—federal law (United States & Canada)

ANTI-EPILEPTICS (e.g., Neurontin)

This class of drugs is usually used to treat epileptic seizures, but they are also widely used as an adjunct to treat various conditions with severe chronic pain. Many of these drugs work by increasing nerve transmission or by blocking certain channels involved in nerve transmission. They are structurally related to the neurotransmitter GABA. Neurontin/gabapentin and Lyrica/Pregabalin are examples of this class of medications.

ANTIDEPRESSANT MEDICATION

Reactive depression can be a part of any chronic illness. Chronic fatigue syndrome and fibromyalgia are no exception. Antidepressants have received a lot of negative press lately, but there is a time and a place for each modality. If all of the other modalities have failed, including talking therapy of some kind like cognitive behavioral therapy, supportive counseling, a trial of therapeutic dose of omega-3 fish oil, etc., and the patient is severely depressed, a trial of antidepressants might help the patient cope with their severe depression. Antidepressants help give patients time to sort out emotional reaction. The same advice—start low and go slow—is applicable for this group of medications. Also, adverse reactions may occur with these drugs, and you should know what to expect before you start them. Any medication can have a paradoxical reaction or the opposite reaction to what is expected. So if you feel *more* depressed when you start an antidepressant, stop taking it and phone your doctor immediately. If the doctor is not available, go immediately to the emergency room and get some medical help.

If the antidepressants are not successful and the patient is suicidal the patient must be admitted voluntarily or committed to a hospital for treatment to prevent suicide. Suicide is a permanent solution to a temporary problem. Most, but not all, episodes of depression eventually improve on their own, even if left untreated. However, many patients do not have the coping skills or energy to ride it out and can benefit dramatically from the cor-

REMEMBER, SUICIDE IS A
PERMANENT SOLUTION
TO A **TEMPORARY PROBLEM.**

rect type and dose of antidepressant. Patients do commit suicide as a result of these illnesses. It is more common than you think. Often it is associated with being poor, isolated, depressed, and worst of all in chronic pain, either undertreated or untreatable pain. Suicide is devastating to the patient's family and friends, who usually just didn't realize "how bad it was."

So please—if you are depressed or in severe pain go for help now. Don't give up! Phone a suicide crisis help line. If you don't know the number, phone the operator. She will call for you. Help is a phone call away. Believe it! Remember, suicide is a permanent solution to a temporary problem.

Tricyclic Antidepressants (TCAs, e.g., Amitriptyline, Doxepin)

Most drugs in this category work by increasing the concentration of certain brain neurotransmitters, specifically serotonin and/or norepinephrine (also known as noradrenaline), by blocking their reuptake by nerve cells in the brain. They are helpful for treating the reactive depression many CFS/FM patients suffer from, called *reactive* because the depression occurs as a reaction to being chronically ill. They may also be prescribed solely for pain relief, especially with fibromyalgia.

Serotonin is a well-known neurotransmitter that helps regulate mood, pain, and sleep. Research has found that patients with CFS/FM poorly process serotonin or have low levels of it. Decreased serotonin levels may lead to alterations in substance P (a hormone involved in the pain response) and deep, delta-wave sleep cycles, which may be one of the reasons FM sufferers experience widespread pain. Abnormal processing of serotonin may also be the reason why CFS/FM sufferers have a lack of restorative deep sleep. Sleep is not only about quantity, *high-quality* sleep is essential in the production of certain growth hormones that repair and restore muscles. Furthermore, serotonin increases the efficiency of endorphins, the body's natural painkillers. TCAs also have the ability to affect other brain neurotransmitter channels involved in the pain response. Studies have shown that TCAs are beneficial in treating some of the associated syndromes of CFS/FM, such as irritable bowel syndrome, temporomandibular joint syndrome, and chronic low back pain, as well as in the prevention of recurrent chronic tension–type headaches.

Selective Serotonin Reuptake Inhibitors (SSRIs, e.g., Paxil, Zoloft)

These drugs work in a similar fashion to TCAs in that they increase the concentration of serotonin in the brain. However, they often have fewer side effects than TCAs because, as their name suggests, they specifically block the reuptake of serotonin in the brain's nerve cells and don't affect the other brain neurotransmitters. A concern for some CFS/FM patients is that SSRIs may worsen sleep disturbances, as one of their potential side effects is insomnia. Therefore it is best to take them first thing in the morning, and for some patients, TCAs may be a better option in any case. It is ultimately dependent upon the individual's reactions to the medication. However, SSRIs are very effective in regulating mood. Indeed, SSRIs are widely used in the field of psychiatry for the following uses: depression, anxiety, and phobias. Like TCAs, SSRIs may also help to prevent the recurrence of chronic tension–type headaches.

Dual Reuptake Inhibitors (DRIs, e.g., Effexor)

Like TCAs, these drugs increase the concentration of both serotonin and norepinephrine in the brain by blocking their reuptake by nerve cells. However, unlike TCAs, DRIs don't affect other brain neurotransmitter systems; therefore, they have fewer side effects. Venlafaxine/Effexor is the only DRI currently available in the Unites States and Canada. A study has shown that it is effective in preventing migraines and tension headaches, and in high doses it can treat multiple symptoms of FM. Milnacipran is a DRI only available in Europe and Japan. It is in development in the United States for the treatment of FM, since studies have shown that it improves pain, fatigue, mood, and sleep in these patients.

MEDICATION TO HELP LOW BLOOD PRESSURE

Adrenergic Drugs

This class of drugs contains commonly prescribed heart medications. In CFS/FM they are used to treat low blood pressure and elevated heart rate. These symptoms are likely related to the body's low blood volume and the difficulty with regulating the autonomic nervous system associated with the function of the heart. Adrenergic drugs can alter nerve transmission in pathways involved in the regulation of blood pressure, heart rate, and the diameter of bronchi. They are used to treat CFS/FM patients in an effort to address low blood pressure when standing (orthostatic hypotension), low blood pressure when standing with an irregular heart rate (postural orthostatic tachycardia syndrome, or POTS), and dizziness. Alpha-adrenergic agonists help to prevent orthostatic hypotension and dizziness by making the diameter of veins smaller, which helps to prevent too much blood from pooling in the lower body when you stand. Beta-adrenergic agonists (better known as beta blockers) can help to regulate orthostatic blood pressure and heart rate in POTS by reducing heart rate and by increasing the filling time of the heart.

Glucocorticoids (e.g., Florinef)

Fludrocortisone is a corticosteroid (or glucocorticoid) that has not been found to be effective when used on its own, but when it is combined with alpha-adrenergic agonists or beta-blockers, it has sometimes been found to be effective in the treatment of orthostatic hypotension, POTS, or dizziness. This drug works by increasing the amount of sodium and water in the body. Two studies have shown that short-term, low-dose use of corticosteroids provided some improvement in fatigue. This is a case where clinical experience and the individual presentation of CFS/FM symptoms will help your doctor determine an appropriate dose. Long-term use has not clinically shown to be very effective in my experience.

IMMUNE DYSFUNCTION MEDICATION

Immune Stimulator and Viral Modulator

Although the cause of CFS is not known, research suggests that a dysfunction of the immune system, often started by a viral infection, may play an important role in this condition. Therefore, immune stimulators and viral modulators, such as Ampligen, are sometimes prescribed. It is usually prescribed to CFS patients with abnormalities in enzyme systems that are involved in immune and antiviral activities in the body. Studies have shown that Ampligen can produce improvements in exercise capacity, memory and cognitive ability, and activities of daily living, and lead to a reduction in visits to health care providers. Ampligen is not routinely prescribed to most patients as it is currently only available in an intravenous product form.

In addition, new research suggests that Valtrex/valcyclovir may be of benefit in CFS by limiting replication of the herpes family viruses. A recent trial demonstrated that Valtrex is effective in limiting the replication of Epstein-Barr virus (EBV) in a four-month controlled study. This is significant because CFS/FM patients often have high EBV antibodies and, at least for some, the reactivation of EBV may contribute to symptoms and the course of the illness.

Imunovir (isoprinosine) is another medication that is being studied in the treatment of CFS. Clinical improvement in chronic fatigue syndrome has been associated with enhanced natural killer cell–mediated cytotoxicity (*Journal of Chronic*

Fatigue Syndrome, 2003). A larger Phase II drug trial investigating its effects in CFS patients is ongoing as of this writing.

INFECTIONS

The use of antibiotic therapy is indicated for the treatment of infections. In my experience some patients have infections that can be difficult to diagnose. They may be bacterial infections in the urinary bladder, ongoing dental infections, or chronic sinus and bronchitis infections, to name a few. Some of these infections, such as HHV6 and mycoplasma, may need special tests such as PCR testing, which may not always be available in some medical systems (for example, Canada).

One especially difficult infection to diagnose is chronic Lyme disease. The diagnosis of chronic Lyme disease by specialized Western blot testing is also indicated if the patient has potentially been exposed to tics that carry the Lyme spirochete. This is a difficult area of medicine at the moment because the diagnosis of chronic Lyme disease is complicated even when this special testing is done in the laboratory. The testing is not straightforward. This is an entire subject by itself in an evolving field of medicine called infectious disease. From my common sense viewpoint, it makes sense to me that if syphilis, which is a spirochete, can have chronic forms (and we know it can), then why can't Lyme disease have a chronic form? I'll leave this subject to others much more knowledgeable than myself.

FUTURE DIRECTIONS

The following drug category is not widely used to treat CFS/FM, but a few studies have shown these medications may provide some benefit. Because this class of drugs is currently available only in Europe, I have no personal experience with it.

5-HT3 Antagonists (e.g., Navoban, Zofran)

This class of drug blocks serotonin type 3 receptors and is normally used to treat nausea and vomiting due to chemotherapy.

Tropisetron is one such drug that has been tested extensively in Europe for the treatment of FM patients, but it is not available in the United States or Canada. One study found that it effectively treats pain, sleep, fatigue, and mood in FM patients. A second study showed that using a low-dose of tropisetron in FM sufferers for ten days resulted in decreased pain intensity and number of painful tender points that lasted even twelve months after the trial was over, and its effects were better than that of both placebo and higher doses of the drug.

Table 1. Antidepressants (generics are shown in regular type, brand names in italics).

Tricyclics (TCAs)
Examples: Amitriptyline hydrochloride *(Elavil, Endep)*, Doxepin *(Sinequan, Adapin)*, Nortriptyline *(Pamelor, Aventyl)*.
Clinical uses for CFS/FM patients: pain relief, sleep disturbances, irritable bowel syndrome, temporomandibular joint syndrome, chronic low back pain, and the prevention of recurrent tension-type headaches.
Possible side effects: increased appetite, constipation, difficulty concentrating, dizziness, daytime drowsiness, dry mouth, headache, nausea, sleep disturbances, tiredness, unpleasant taste, urinary retention, weakness, weight gain.

Selective Serotonin Reuptake Inhibitors (SSRIs)
Examples: Fluoxetine *(Prozac)*, Sertraline *(Zoloft)*, Paroxetine *(Paxil)*.
Clinical uses for CFS/FM patients: mood disorders and the prevention of recurrent tension-type headaches; for individuals who cannot tolerate the side-effects of TCAs.
Possible side effects: insomnia or difficulty sleeping, dry mouth, headache, decreased sexual drive or ability, dizziness, diarrhea or constipation, weight gain.

Table 1 (continued).

Dual Reuptake Inhibitors (DRIs)
Examples: Venlafaxine *(Effexor)*, Milnacipran *(Ixel)*, Duloxetine *(Cymbalta)*.
Clinical uses for CFS/FM patients: the prevention of migraines and tension-type headaches and treatment of multiple symptoms in FM patients such as pain, fatigue, mood, and sleep.
Possible side effects: increased blood pressure, anorexia, constipation, decreased strength, dizziness, drowsiness, dry mouth, ejaculation problems, impotence, nervousness, sweating.

Norepinephrine (Noradrenaline) Reuptake Inhibitors (NRIs)
Examples: Reboxetine (Edronax, Vestra).
Clinical uses for CFS/FM patients: pain and fatigue found in FM sufferers.
Possible side effects: dry mouth, constipation, impotence, insomnia, increased sweating, rapid heart beat, urinary retention, vertigo.

Table 2. Non-steriodal anti-inflammatory drugs (NSAIDs).

NSAIDs
Examples: Aspirin *(Anacin, Ascriptin, Bayer, Ecotrin, Excedrin tablets, ZORprin)*, Ibuprofen *(Advil, Motrin, Mediprin, Nuprin)*, Ketoprofen *(Actron, Orudis KT)*, Naproxen sodium *(Aleve)*.
Clinical uses for CFS/FM patients: pain relief for concomitant osteoarthritis, rheumatoid arthritis, or chronic low back pain.
Possible side effects: abdominal pain, chronic daily headaches, fluid retention, gastric ulcers, gastric bleeding, increased risk of bleeding or bruising from cuts, heartburn, indigestion, lightheadedness, nausea, decreased kidney function, increased liver enzymes.

COX-2 Inhibitors
Examples: Celecoxib *(Celebrex)*, Rofecoxib *(Vioxx)*.
Clinical uses for CFS/FM patients: same as above.
Possible side effects: same as above, but there is a lower risk of stomach upset or stomach ulcers. Possible increased risk of heart attack and stroke.

Table 3. Analgesics.

Acetaminophen

Examples: Acetaminophen *(aspirin-free Anacin, Excedrin caplets, Panadol, Tylenol)*, Acetaminophen with codeine *(Fiorcet, Phenaphen with codeine, Tylenol with codeine)*.

Clinical uses for CFS/FM patients: minor pain relief.

Possible side effects: long-term use may lead to liver damage when used with other substances that can damage the liver such as alcohol. Acetaminophen with codeine can lead to constipation, dizziness, drowsiness, tiredness, vomiting.

Tramadol Hydrochloride

Examples: *Ultram.*

Clinical uses for CFS/FM patients: pain relief, chronic daily headaches, low back pain.

Possible side effects: anxiety, blurred vision, constipation, dependency, diarrhea, dizziness, drowsiness, headache, nausea, nervousness, sleep disturbances, upset stomach, vomiting.

Narcotics

Examples: Codeine (usually combined with *Tylenol*), Hydrocodone with acetominophen *(Percoset, Dolacet, Hydrocet, Lorcet, Lortab, Vicodin)*, Oxycodone *(OxyContin, Roxicodone)*, Meperidine *(Demerol)*, Morphine *(Astramorph PF, Duramorph, Infumorph, Kadian, MS Contin, Hydromorph Contin, Oramorph SR, Roxanol, Roxanol Rescudose)*, Propoxyphene hydrochloride *(Darvon, PC-Cap, Wygesic)*, Fentanyl *(duragesic patch)*.

Clinical uses for CFS/FM patients: pain relief.

Possible side effects: constipation, dependency, dizziness, drowsiness, itching, tolerance, nausea, weakness, vomiting; at very high doses, respiratory depression and death.

Table 4. Benzodiazepines/sleep medications.

Examples: Clonazepam *(Klonopin)*, Diazepam *(Valium)*, Lorazepam *(Ativan)*, Nitrazepam *(Mogadon)*; Non-benzodiazepine hypnotics: Zalepon *(Sonata)*, Zolpidem *(Stillnoct)*, Zopiclone *(Imovane)*, Trazodone *(Desyrel)*.
Clinical uses for CFS/FM patients: anxiety, insomnia, fatigue.
Possible side effects: addiction, aggression, confusion, dependence, drowsiness, enhanced effects of alcohol, morning "hang-over," light-headedness, memory loss, tolerance.

Table 5. CNS stimulants.

Examples: Methylphenidate *(Ritalin, Concerta, Methylin)*, Dexamphetamine *(Dexedrine, Adderall)*, Modafinil *(Provigil)*.
Clinical uses for CFS/FM patients: to increase energy and alertness.
Possible side effects: addiction, anorexia, anxiety, dizziness, dry mouth, headache, irritability, nausea, nervousness, tolerance, worsening of sleep disorders.

Table 6. Adrenergic drugs/low blood pressure medications.

Alpha-Adrenergic Agonists
Examples: Midodrine *(ProAmatine)*.
Clinical uses for CFS/FM patients: orthostatic hypotension and dizziness.
Possible side effects: abnormal heart rate, decreased heart rate, decreased urination, headache, increased blood pressure while lying down, itchy skin.

Beta-Adrenergic Antagonists
Examples: Pindolol *(Visken)*, Atenolol *(Tenormin)*.
Clinical uses for CFS/FM patients: orthostatic hypotension, dizziness, postural orthostatic tachycardia syndrome.
Possible side effects: constipation, decreased heart rate, diarrhea, drowsiness, headache, insomnia, spasms of the bronchi, tiredness, worsening of orthostatic hypotension.

Table 7. Blood pressure/glucocorticoids.

Examples: Fludrocortisone *(Florinef)*, Cortisone *(Cortone)*, Prednisone *(Cortan, Deltasone, Meticorten, Orasone)*.
Clinical uses for CFS/FM patients: Fludrocortisone can be used in combination with alpha-adrenergic agonists or beta-blockers to treat orthostatic hypotension, POTS, or dizziness; most corticosteroids are used to treat pain and studies have shown benefit for treating fatigue.
Possible side effects: acne, anxiety, depression, dizziness, headache, insomnia, irregular menstrual periods, restlessness, upset stomach, vomiting, weight gain.

Table 8. Immune stimulators and viral modulators.

Examples: poly I: poly C12U *(Ampligen)*, Acyclovir, *Valtrex*.
Clinical uses for CFS/FM patients: improved exercise capacity, memory and cognitive ability, activities of daily living, fewer emergency room and hospital visits.
Possible side effects: flu-like symptoms, flushing of the face, headaches, light-headedness, swollen glands.

Table 9. Muscle relaxants.

Cyclobenzaprine
Examples: Cyclobenzaprine.
Clinical uses for CFS/FM patients: pain, sleep disorders, irritable bowel syndrome, fatigue, reducing the number of painful trigger points.
Possible side effects: blurred vision, dizziness, drowsiness, dry mouth, fatigue, unpleasant taste.

Tizanidine
Examples: Tizanidine *(Zanaflex)*.
Clinical uses for CFS/FM patients: chronic daily headaches, low back pain, sleep, pain.
Possible side effects: dizziness, drowsiness, dry mouth, light-headedness upon standing, increased liver enzymes, tiredness, unsteadiness, vision problems, weakness, yellowing of the skin.

Table 10. Other drugs.

5-HT3 Antagonists
Examples: Tropisetron *(Navoban).*
Clinical uses for CFS/FM patients: pain, sleep, fatigue, mood, reducing the number of painful tender points.
Possible side effects: constipation, diarrhea, dizziness, headache, loss of appetite, stomach pain, tiredness.

NMDA Antagonists for Pain
Examples: Ketamine *(Ketalar),* Amantadine *(Symmetrel),* Methadone *(Physeptone).*
Clinical uses for CFS/FM patients: pain.
Possible side effects: blurred vision, confusion, constipation, decreased energy, drowsiness, dry mouth, forgetfulness, irritability, nausea, vomiting.

Growth Hormone
Examples: *Saizen, Zomacton.*
Clinical uses for CFS/FM patients: pain, sleep, fatigue, reducing the number of tender points in FM patients.
Possible side effects: worsening of symptoms.

Anti-Epileptics for Pain
Examples: Pregabalin, Neurontin *(Gabapentin),* Clonazepam *(Klonopin, Rivortil).*
Clinical uses for CFS/FM patients: pain, sleep disturbances, fatigue, recurring headaches, temporomandibular joint syndrome, restless leg syndrome, anxiety.
Possible side effects: anxiety, blurred vision, drowsiness, fatigue, headache, irregular eye movements, tremor.

CHAPTER SUMMARY

- The use of medications in CFS/FM is not an exact science. Physicians will work with patients individually trying different medications to determine which medication is most effective.
- Due to the sensitivities of CFS/FM patients, your doctor may have to start with extremely low doses of medications and work up slowly as tolerated.
- Medications are not a cure for CFS/FM; they are currently used as a supportive intervention to reduce symptoms.
- A wide range of drug classes may have therapeutic potential in CFS/FM.
- Remain hopeful because research scientists are hard at work determining if new medications may be valuable.

CHAPTER NINE

LEGAL SUPPORT

Chronic fatigue syndrome and fibromyalgia patients often may be so ill that they can no longer carry out their normal occupations, and the effect can be devastating on the individuals and their families. People of all ages, educational backgrounds, and social standings, and of both genders, have been struck by these illnesses to such an extent that they can no longer work. Besides the impact on the individual's self-esteem, mental health, and familial relationships, the cold, hard economic reality also comes into play. An individual who is too ill to work can suffer from a significant reduction in income, lifestyle, and the ability to obtain much-needed medical care. Unfortunately, when individuals with CFS/FM are at their worst, they are then forced into hostile interactions with different income replacement systems, a stressor they are not often equipped to deal with. Fatigue, pain, and associated cognitive difficulties reduce the individual's abil-

HERMAN®

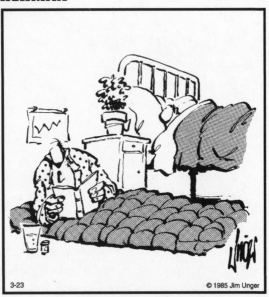

3-23   © 1985 Jim Unger

**"Twelve years I've been paying
into that medical plan."**

ity to deal with the administrative systems they desperately need to access when forced to leave an occupation. The main focus of this chapter will be the utilization of the legal system in an effort to secure financial security. However, some patients may use the advice to secure a working environment accommodated to their particular needs.

Many government agencies and almost all private insurers seem rather skeptical about the origins and impact of CFS/FM. The questions of whether the illness actually exists, and whether its symptoms are disabling, both in general and in specific cases, are often disputed. Agencies and insurers often reject claims for income replacement made by CFS/FM patients out of hand. This sets up the CFS/FM patient for a conflict, at the time when they have the least amount of resources, financial and personal, to carry out this fight. Finding and retaining appropriate legal assistance at this point can be crucial to your success or failure to maintain economic stability over what may be a very long and painful illness.

WHEN YOU NEED A LAWYER

When attempting to replace your income, a lawyer is usually not required for the initial application process either to a government plan or private insurer. Unless the claim forms are particularly complex or require the signature of a commissioner or a notary, there is no need to engage a lawyer for the initial preparation and delivery of paperwork to the insurer. To be frank, nobody knows the facts of your medical condition and personal life like you do, and a lawyer can add little to this part of the process. Assuming you are able to complete the forms on your own and your doctor is cooperative in providing the normally requested medical analysis at the opening of the file, retaining a lawyer for the initial application may simply be a waste of your precious funds.

A lawyer becomes important when the government agency or the insurer has refused your claim. Once they have indicated in writing that they are not willing to pay your claim, the situation has changed greatly. The government agency or insurer is no longer investigating your claim, they have rendered a decision that has made them adversarial to you. To put it simply you have requested that they pay you, they have decided they are not going to, and they are likely to stand behind this decision unless they are forced by legal means to change their stance.

Once the clear refusal of your claim has been received, it is time to consult with and likely retain a lawyer to assist you in pursuing your income replacement benefits. At this point in the process, no delay should be allowed to occur. In almost every jurisdiction there are time limits known as "limitation periods," which must be strictly adhered to. In other words, if you do not move quickly in challenging the refusal of the government agency or the insurer, you may permanently lose your right to do so. While every jurisdiction has different time periods available to claimants, none of them allow an indefinite period of time to bring suit to force payment of duly owed benefits. Every day that passes after you received the negative decision from the agency or insurer is one day closer to the ultimate limitation period when you will no longer be able to pursue this claim successfully. The documents delivered to you from the government agency or the insurer do not always make the limitation period for your case clear. You should immediately consult with a qualified legal counsel after receiving rejection from the agency/insurer, and one of your first questions to that lawyer should be, "How long do I have to bring suit on my claim?"

HOW TO FIND A LAWYER

Looking for counsel to represent you in a long-term disability claim is not as simple as going to the Yellow Pages. It is likely that you will have a relationship of some years with this lawyer, and you will be entrusting him to deliver you an appropriate result to protect your future and that of your family over a potentially lengthy illness. Choosing the right lawyer to represent you on a long-term disability matter is one of the most important decisions you may make in your lifetime. You should treat it that way.

The best way to seek out a lawyer to represent you in a claim of this nature will be from a direct word-of-mouth referral. Perhaps someone you know from a support group or a chat-room, or another CFS/FM patient you have met, has fought a similar battle and has had very good results with a lawyer they speak well of. If you do not have an acquaintance who can assist you in this way, one of the doctors who treat you for this illness may have a recommendation for you. Often doctors will have served as witnesses or been in touch with lawyers over the course of claims, and they may be able to tell you the name of an individual they found competent and efficient to deal with. Most doctors deal with a number of lawyers over the course of their careers, thus becoming fairly experienced in what to expect from a quality lawyer. Their advice can be invaluable to you.

If you are unable to find a personal referral to a lawyer, then the next logical step is to contact your local Trial Lawyers Association. In addition to national trial lawyers groups, each American state and most of Canada's provinces have an organization of trial lawyers who work in the area of personal injury litigation. The national body in the United States is the American Trial Lawyers Association, and the largest similar body in Canada is the Ontario Trial Lawyers Association. Once you contact these organizations, you can ask them for a referral to a lawyer who does long-term disability work and has experience with CFS/FM. You may also inquire as to whether they have a study group designed to enhance their litigation skills in long-term disability litigation, as the Ontario Trial Lawyers Association does. If they have a group dedicated to the study and enhancement of their skills in this area, it only makes sense to ask the Trial Lawyers Association for the names of the lawyers closest to you who are members of that group. While retaining a member of a Trial Lawyers Association is not a guarantee of success or perfect quality in your counsel, it is certainly a lot better than simply selecting a name out of the Yellow Pages or based on a flashy ad.

What to Look for in a Lawyer

Once you are in the lawyer's office, there are a number of areas you should review with him before making a final decision whether or not the lawyer is right to represent your case. You are perfectly entitled to visit with several lawyers before you make your decision to find the lawyer who best suits your needs. No lawyer should take this process personally. Here are some areas that should be carefully considered before you make a decision on which lawyer to retain:

1. Experience in long-term disability cases—While these cases may not be incredibly different from other types of contract and personal injury litigation, they do have a number of nuances of their own, and a lawyer with the most specific expertise possible will be able to get better results for you.

2. Experience with CFS/FM cases—Even today, CFS/FM are not well understood in the legal community. There is a battery of articles and medical information required to be understood to effectively present the CFS/FM case. The more experienced your lawyer is with these illnesses, the more he or she will be able to represent you effectively.

3. Sound medical knowledge—The lawyer you retain should already have a base knowledge of CFS/FM and related ailments. By asking a few simple questions or listening closely to the lawyer in the initial interview, you should be able to determine whether he is familiar with the literature in the field. You would rather retain somebody who already has the information than pay someone to learn it from the bottom up.

4. Contingency fee retainers—Almost every jurisdiction in the United States and Canada allows a lawyer to take matters on a contingency fee—that is, an arrangement that is paid based on the amount of funds they recover for you.

Conducting litigation over a number of years can be a very expensive process, and if you are unable to work, it is unlikely you will be able to pay ongoing hourly rates. Lawyers who are familiar with this field operate on a contingency basis in a standard fashion.

5. Adequate staff—Long-term disability and personal injury files require a great deal of labor to ensure that medical records, court records, and other documents are properly organized. Consider that lawyers are often not available to return your call, and it is often their staff that will do so. A lawyer with a small staff may not be able to give your file the attention it requires or return your calls or request for information as promptly as he or she might otherwise be able to.

6. Plain English communication—The lawyer you deal with should be able to translate complex legal concepts into layperson's terms so you can understand it. The ultimate decision-maker in any lawsuit is the client. Lawyers who use complex language or legalese in order to impress people are doing their clients a disservice by not communicating effectively. Find a lawyer who understands the importance of communicating in straightforward language.

7. Patience—Individuals with CFS/FM often suffer from cognitive impairments and ask questions more than once. They occasionally need things explained a number of times until the information sinks through their brain fog so they can understand it. This requires some patience on the part of the lawyer, and, sadly, not all have this quality.

8. An appropriate expert database—The lawyer should have a number of medical-legal experts who are familiar with CFS/FM to whom they will refer you over the course of building the claim. Certain doctors have the appropriate qualifications and background to provide effective reports when a lawyer is building a claim for long-term disability. Quite often, using your treating doctor is not enough; it is

important to find a lawyer who has an effective data base of medical-legal experts qualified to testify on your behalf.

9. Membership in appropriate Trial Lawyers Association—While this is not a guarantee of any sort, it shows the lawyer is serious about the work he or she does and dedicated to continuing education and becoming a more effective counsel.

10. Good "fit"—A lawyer is like any other human being. Some of them you will get along with; some of them you will not. Their communication style may be very effective with you, or it may not. Or you may find that you just do not particularly like the person. Considering you will be dealing with this lawyer over a number of years, it is important to find someone with a personality that you can work with. No lawyer should be insulted if you choose not to retain them on any basis; thus, carefully assess whether you think you would enjoy working with that lawyer over a period of some years.

What to Expect from Your Lawyer

1. Aggressive representation—A lawyer should believe in your case and advocate for you aggressively. It is a well-known maxim that litigation is not a tea party, and your lawyer should be willing to fight for your rights in an aggressive fashion. This is a basic feature of any successful litigation lawyer, and he or she should not be willing to compromise on this issue.

2. Appropriate medical-legal referrals—Over the course of your claim, your lawyer should send you to appropriate doctors and other experts who assist in building your case. In most situations your lawyer will fund these referrals until the end of the case.

3. Reasonable communications—Your lawyer should be willing to respond to reasonable requests for the status of your action. While you may not always be satisfied with the

speed of your action or the progress of your matter, it should not be difficult to find out what is going on with your case at any particular time. Phone calls should be returned by a lawyer or a staff member within a reasonable time frame.

4. Courtesy—All professionals should treat you with courtesy; lawyers should be no exception.

5. Open door policy—The lawyer should make himself available for a reasonable number of appointments when you need to speak to him. Many of the questions you may have may not be appropriate for his staff to answer, and access to your lawyer within a reasonable period of time should be part of the service offered. Do not be surprised, however, if you have to wait two or three weeks for an appointment with your counsel—or perhaps even longer in the event he or she is engaged in a trial at the time you call.

6. Open file policy—The contents of your file are effectively your property. You should be able to get copies of documents and other information from your file after a reasonable time has elapsed.

7. Clear time tables—The litigation process, while it varies from case to case, usually follows within certain formats. Your lawyer should be able to give you some guidance as to the speed and timing of your case so that you can make appropriate arrangements to live your life in the interim. While you may not like what your lawyer tells you about the timing of the justice system in your jurisdiction, he or she should be able to explain it to you in a fairly straightforward fashion. Delay should also be explained to you by your counsel as well.

8. Honesty—This is a deal breaker. The lawyer should always be honest with you. If you find your lawyer has been dishonest with you, you should seek new counsel immediately.

9. Faith in your case—It requires a certain amount of spirit and energy to prosecute a case effectively. If you conclude that your lawyer does not have faith in the justice of your

case or the success of your case, you should make inquiries with your lawyer about his or her commitment level to your case immediately. If you are not convinced that your lawyer believes in your case enough to prosecute it effectively, you should seek new counsel.

10. Clear settlement advice—You should not simply accept a lawyer's opinion on why a settlement may be good or bad. It is not good enough for a lawyer to say $100,000 is a good settlement. He or she must be able to explain to you why any offer or proposal is a good or bad one in any particular case. He or she should take the time to explain to you how the numbers were determined, and assess the risks involved in proceeding or not accepting the offer at all. If a lawyer is not willing or able to explain why an offer is good or bad, it is not an offer that you should accept.

What Not to Expect from Your Lawyer

1. Instant communications—Most litigation lawyers are extremely busy individuals; they service a number of clients and are often required to be in court to argue trials or motions. All your requests for information cannot be answered immediately. Even if you are able to get the appropriate staff member on the phone, he or she may have to go to your file to obtain documents to answer your question or make inquiries of the lawyer to give you an effective answer. This may result in some delay in getting answers to your questions but will likely result in your getting better answers to your questions rather than a flip answer without the facts being checked.

2. Perfect knowledge of your case—A lawyer represents a number of clients and will not be able to memorize every detail of your case and keep it at his fingertips at all times. While the lawyer should be generally familiar with your case and the facts that are driving it, do not expect him to know your life as well as you do.

3. Psychic ability—Lawyers are not mind-readers. They will
    not understand or know what your concerns are in every
    case until you tell them what they are. Communication is a
    two-way street. It is the obligation of the lawyer to try and
    communicate as effectively as possible with you and give
    you the information you need to understand your situation.
    On the other hand, it is your obligation to ask the lawyer
    questions in areas you do not feel she has explained ade-
    quately and make it clear to the lawyer when you feel she
    has not communicated clearly enough with you.
4. Rapid results—The litigation system in almost every jurisdic-
    tion is slow. Cases can take years from inception to the time
    they get to trial. While every client feels their case is the
    most dire and desperate, it is very difficult to force the courts
    to expedite the hearing of any particular case. The wheels of
    justice in North America turn slowly, and this is a reality that
    you will have to live with over the course of the litigation.
5. Blind obedience—Your lawyer is an independent profes-
    sional who has certain ethical duties he must fulfill. He
    cannot follow all of your instructions blindly. He may not
    be able to do exactly as you tell him, as it may cause him to
    breach one of his ethical duties. He has certain professional
    concerns related to his reputation and respect among fellow
    members of the bar as well. You may wish to give instruc-
    tions that you feel advance your case. However, if your
    lawyer believes it will either damage his own reputation,
    cause an ethical breach, or weaken his credibility as your
    advocate, he will decline to follow some instructions. You
    should take his advice in this area very seriously before you
    consider changing to another lawyer.

What a Lawyer Should Expect from You

1. Honesty—This is a deal breaker both ways. A dishonest
    client can only bring a lawyer grief and embarrassment. You
    need to be open and honest with your lawyer at all times so

she can assess your case fully. There are few problems a
skilled lawyer cannot overcome, but she cannot solve problems if you fail to disclose them.

2. Organization—You will often be providing significant
   amounts of information and documents to your lawyer.
   Anything you can do to organize this material before you
   deliver it to the lawyer in some chronological or topical
   fashion will assist your counsel in representing you. It will
   also save you money, as the lawyer and her staff will have to
   spend less time reorganizing your documentation.

3. Prompt response to communications—Occasionally, your
   lawyer will need information from you on a prompt basis;
   you should strive to provide it accordingly.

4. Full cooperation in the process—Occasionally your counsel
   will recommend that you go to medical-legal assessments or
   discoveries or be involved in motions or other proceedings
   that he or she believes adds tactical value to your case. It is
   impossible for your lawyer to educate you fully in the many
   nuances of effective disability litigation so to some degree
   you need to have faith in her opinion so that your case can
   move forward.

5. Courtesy to the staff—You may become frustrated and angry
   over the length of time a matter is taking and the impact it
   is having on you and your family. However, there is never
   an excuse to be discourteous, rude, or aggressive to a member of your lawyer's staff, no matter what you think of the
   situation at the time.

6. Faith in your counsel's opinion—While you should not follow his opinion blindly, hopefully you will have built up a
   degree of confidence in your lawyer that will give you faith
   in his opinion. He will be giving you advice that will have
   significant impact on the outcome of your case, which can
   change the course of your entire life. If you do not have
   faith in your lawyer's opinion, this is not a lawyer you
   should be dealing with.

7. Patience—The justice system is a slow one. While you may find it taxing at times, if you are patient and your lawyer moves the matter appropriately, you will get a just result. Being impatient and trying to force matters when they are not ready to be moved forward can result in a negative outcome for you.

8. Complete disclosure—Your lawyer needs to hear all the information that might be relevant to your case and receive all the documents from you that may be relevant to your case. It is not your job to decide which documents are relevant to the case and which are not. It is always the best policy to give your lawyer as much information and documentation as possible and let him decide whether or not, or how, the information will be used in advancing your matter.

9. Questions—When a client asks a lawyer a lot of questions, the lawyer understands that the client is fully engaged in the case, has certain concerns, and is giving her the opportunity to fill in the blanks that the client needs to have filled in. It is the client who never seems to ask questions that makes lawyers nervous, as it is hard to tell whether or not they have given the client the information they require or have effectively answered that client's concerns.

10. Reasonable instructions—While you may have a great deal of anger and resentment about how you have been treated by your insurer or government agency in rejecting your claim, anger is not an effective basis from which to make decisions in your litigation. Your lawyer needs directions from you on how to handle proposals and how to resolve the matter, and if you simply allow your anger and emotion to rule, you will not be able to give your lawyer effective instructions. No matter how hard it may be, you really need to put aside some of the anger resulting from the situation so that you can make appropriate decisions. Your lawyer

cannot be an advocate for you if you cannot give him effective, clear-headed direction.

DISABILITY COVERAGE

It is important that you canvass all types of coverage available to help replace your income for the time you are going to be off work. There are often a number of systems available to assist you in any jurisdiction, including government agencies and programs, work disability insurance plans, and private disability insurance plans. While it is impossible to cover the details of each jurisdiction in a book of this nature, you need to be incredibly thorough in asking questions and making inquiries of all the relevant government agencies, your employer, and any insurer that you have had dealings with over the years. As an example, an individual in Ontario may have coverage available to them while they are disabled from any of the following sources, and perhaps more;

- Canada Pension Plan Disability Benefits
- Ontario Disability Support Plan
- Ontario Works Program
- Group Disability Insurance
- Private Disability Insurance
- Credit Disability Insurance
- Mortgage Disability Insurance
- Union or Fraternal Organization Insurance
- Alumni Insurance through University

You must be extremely thorough in canvassing all of these areas so you can ensure that the economic impact on yourself and your family will be the minimum possible while you are off work and that you are receiving all the benefits to which you are entitled under the various plans and policies.

Types of Disability Policies

There are many types of disability policies available to individuals. There are group policies, private policies, taxable policies, and nontaxable policies. Many of them have a series of different definitions to deal with including questions about what constitutes a disability and what constitutes regular medical care. However, for the purposes of a doctor trying to help a patient deal with her disability insurer or an insured making an application, most of these distinctions are irrelevant. The only substantial concern for medical practitioners is whether the policy calls for a definition of disability based on "own occupation" or one based on "any occupation." The letter from the insurer asking for a report or an opinion should set out which of the two "occupations" is being addressed. In the event the insurer has not provided your treatment provider with information, you can request it from your insurer before they deliver their opinion. As you will see from the remaining discussion, the border between these two definitions has substantial overlap that will often allow your doctor to write an effective opinion even without knowing which type of policy is in place.

"Own Occupation" Policies

If the insured has an "own occupation" policy, he is entitled to benefits so long as he is unable to resume his regular occupation. Usually, this refers to the occupation the insured was engaged in at the time he became disabled. Total disability does not require complete helplessness, so the insured can collect benefits if he is "unable to perform all the substantial and material acts required in his usual occupations."

The insured is disabled if a reasonable person would recognize that he shouldn't work. Sometimes the insured is capable of carrying out the tasks which make up his job, but his performance is hindered by pain, fatigue, or medication. In other cases, medical advice or common sense makes it necessary to cease work in order to effect a cure or prolong the insured's life. Pain alone is not a disabling condition, but there are cases in which extreme or persistent pain makes it impossible for the insured to continue working.

The courts have recognized that some jobs require much greater precision and consistency than others. While impaired performances may be tolerable in some occupations, in others, even a small error can have unacceptable consequences, and an individual with a minor disability will be incapable of performing adequately. Thus, a group home worker with whiplash was held to be totally disabled because episodes of disorientation had resulted in two mistakes in dispensing medications to residents. Many other high precision/low error-tolerance occupations can be easily called to mind.

Often the insured has recovered partially and has begun to assume a role in her business, performing at least some of the tasks of her former occupation. At what point she is able to perform "all the substantial and material acts" which make up that occupation is a question of degree, but the courts tend to be lenient toward the insured. This is especially so where the claimant is self-employed or operates her own business. The courts don't expect the claimant to shut down her business because of an illness or injury. The fact that the insured goes to her usual place of business and does what she can or works through pain in order to keep the business going does not, by itself, establish that she is no longer disabled.

The courts have found, based on this logic, that a restaurant manager was considered to be disabled although he could complete his paperwork and a carpenter could be disabled even though he was able to supervise the renovation of his home. In another case, a businessman was held to be disabled despite the fact that he had arranged financing for his enterprise and completed some documentation.

"Any Occupation" Policies

A typical employer's group insurance policy provides the disabled employee with own occupation benefits for a period of one to three years, followed by a period of long-term disability coverage on an "any occupation" basis. The patient will continue to be entitled to benefits during the "any occupation" period so long as he is prevented from engaging in work for which he is "reasonably suited by training, education, or experience" or work that is suited to his "skill and ability" or some other similar phrase.

The transition from own occupation to any occupation coverage is a key moment in the life of a disability claim. Most insurers will take an aggressive approach to the claim when it reaches this point. They will ask for an update from the claimant's treating physicians, and they may request specialists' reports. The insurer may also exercise their right to have their own physician conduct an examination of the insured, and if they haven't done so already, consult experts in rehabilitation regarding alternative occupations.

A commensurate alternative occupation must be something that is comparable to the insured's former line of work in terms of status and potential earnings. The proposed occupation must be something for which the insured is qualified by virtue of his schooling and work experience.

The proposed job must require some sort of real application or effort on the part of the insured, and a position that "involves the performing of practically no work" will not be considered adequate. In one case, the insured obtained an appointment as postmaster in a small town, but virtually all of the work was done by employees and family members, and the court concluded that the appointment was an occupation in name only.

Remuneration

Often the earning potential of an alternative occupation is less than that of the insured's former work. The proposed job must be "reasonably comparable" to the insured's previous work "in status and reward," but the pay level need not match the income which the insured is accustomed to receiving. A disparity between the income of the two occupations is one factor the court will consider when deciding whether the new occupation is suited to the claimant. The adequacy of the remuneration is a question of degree, and there is no clear rule establishing a point where the discrepancy between the old income and the new is unacceptable.

Nature and Status of the Work

The courts recognize that an alternative occupation must be consistent with the insured's personality and background. Thus the tastes and interests of the insured, as well as the nature and status of the previous work, are important factors. The courts are reluctant to accept that an individual can retrain for work that involves a social context and workplace environment that is foreign to them, particularly when the individual is an older worker or someone who has been involved in a particular line of work for a long time.

There are many cases in which courts have refused to compel people who are accustomed to physical labor or outdoor work to switch to clerical duties or light work in a store or office. Similarly, courts have often rejected the suggestion that professionals, managers, and executives should take on work which involves a reduction in social status or even a new specialty within the same profession.

Where the claimant is a young person with no long-standing commitment to a particular type of employment, judges are more likely to conclude that retraining is appropriate.

Does Part-Time Work Qualify?

Whether only being able to work part time qualifies as being "totally disabled" is more of a legal question than a medical one. However, there have been a number of cases in which the court has found the ability to work only part time still leaves one in a state of "total disability." Therefore, when your doctor writes your reports to insurance companies, he or she should not foreclose the possibility of disability simply because an individual who has returned to work part time may not appear to be "totally disabled" from a medical sense. They may well be in a legal sense. A reasonable guide on the issue of disability (although the cases move all over the map on this particular issue) is that if an individual is making only 65 to 70 percent of the amount they made in their occupation previously, then that person may not be "totally disabled," although they may qualify under some policies as being "residually disabled."

The most effective route for the treating practitioner writing a medical report on this issue would be to quantify as precisely as possible the amount of part-time work being done. Any specifics should be passed on to both the insurer and the counsel to assist them in making an accurate determination of their rights under the policy. Since the insurers appear to inherently distrust people who make claims, independent verification of this information from the treating practitioner will often help arrive at a just conclusion.

In the modern environment of CFS/FM, multiple chemical sensitivity, and other so-called functional somatic syndromes, variability of symptoms is an important factor. The courts have ruled quite clearly that an individual who has variable symptoms and cannot commit to a regular scheduled employment due to those symptoms is totally disabled. The courts have taken a much more "real world" approach than the insurers. In the real world, if an individual cannot commit to some sort of work schedule, it is almost impossible to obtain employment. The case law is clear that the variability of symptoms and inability to commit to a regular working schedule can completely disable an individual on their own, even though the symptoms may allow for part-time work or work at times when the individual is in a period of remission or on a "good day."

Objective Versus Subjective Symptoms

Many insurers will ask the doctors only to report "objective" symptoms of illness. This is inappropriate and probably a bad faith step. I have reviewed a significant number of long-term disability contracts, and I have yet to see one which defines disability in terms of "objective" symptoms. There are a number of cases in the United States, and they seem to be migrating north, that indicate the insurer attempting to import the word "objective" into the disability analysis. Once again, where the contract does not call for it, this represents an act of bad faith against the insured by the insurer, which may be punishable by punitive and exemplary damages.

What this means on a practical basis is that medical practitioners who are reporting to claims adjudicators should forward the information about both objective and subjective symptoms they have observed in their patients. It may be a useful technique to break them down into those two categories and list them in that fashion if it is suitable for their reporting style. However, subjective symptoms should not be downplayed or ignored simply because insurers in their criteria and manuals seem to place a higher value on "objective" symptoms. Consider that in the field of psycho-emotional disability, there are virtually no objective symptoms to deal with. As a practitioner who actually treats individuals, you will be well aware that subjective symptoms are crucial to making an effective diagnosis and putting together a treatment plan. They are equally crucial in the analysis of disability.

While on the subject of subjective symptoms, credibility of the patient is also important. If the doctor has concerns about the credibility of the patient or possesses information that enhances credibility in their office assessment, these should be included in the report to the insurer. For instance, if the individual reports strange variable symptoms or is very reluctant to accept treatment this should be reported. Also, a doctor may wish to report that the individual is someone he or she has known for a long period of time who has a long employment history and is forthright and seems to be very open and honest. It is very difficult for an insurer who is looking at a pile of paper rather than an individual to determine whether that individual is credible in their complaints. One of the pieces of information that a treating practitioner has is a "sense" or "feel" for the patient, and they should be willing to transmit this to the insurer to help with analysis.

The credibility of the treating practitioner is also important. The treating practitioner is not an advocate, but rather is someone who should report to the insurer what they see and what they believe. If they see something and believe something strongly, there is nothing wrong with reporting it in such a fashion. If there are concerns or reservations, these should be reported as well. Only through a full and frank dialogue between medical practitioners, claims adjudicators, and counsel can fairness be arrived at for the people who are trying to obtain assistance from their insurers.

The Name Game

Expert medical evidence is important in any case in which disability is an issue, whether the test is "own occupation" or "any occupation" disability. Although the court will normally hear the testimony of the insured's treating physician(s), as well as that of specialists retained by both sides, a diagnosis is not a prerequisite to a finding of disability. So long as evidence establishes an inability to work, it is not necessary for the insured or her doctors to precisely identify the disabling condition. In a Canadian case in which "eminently qualified experts disagree[d] on the appropriate naming" of the insured's problem, the court found it "unnecessary to label or categorically determine the disease or diseases" in question.

The Good Faith Environment

An insurance contract occupies a special place in our legal system. It is not merely a contract but a contract of the "utmost good faith." The obligation extends both ways to each party. Due to the fact that an insured, when the time to rely upon the contract comes about, cannot switch to any other potential party for indemnification of their losses, a special onus is placed upon the insurer in handling these claims. They must deal with the insured's claim on the basis of the "utmost good faith." This is a complex topic that was considered by the Supreme Court of

Canada in the *Whitten v. Pilot* case. It certainly has the potential to be the subject of an entire paper on its own (and hopefully will be), but for the purposes of this discussion there are two important points to consider.

The first point is that the duty of good faith goes both ways. That is, the insured must deal with the insurer in the "utmost good faith." For your purposes this means that you must give over all of your records when asked to by the insurer. The insured has an obligation to give the insurer full details of the claim and their medical condition in order to allow them to properly assess the claim in its context. In almost every case where it has been requested, the court has ordered that the patient give over the full clinical notes and records of all treating practitioners in a long-term disability case. Not only is resistance of this kind of request futile, it is counterproductive. Insurers operate on a fairly simple response basis. In the event that the treating physician or patient refuses to give up cogent clinical notes and records, then the insurer will automatically assume the patient or claimant is trying to hide something. The duty of "utmost good faith" placed upon the insured requires full cooperation from the patient and the treating practitioner.

The jurisprudence in this area has defined a number of other duties that are the responsibility of the insurer. There are far too many duties to be enumerated here, and in general, they are not a concern in the vast majority of cases. However, it is the duty of the insurer to consider in his decision-making process the impact the decision will have on the condition of the insured. This also includes investigative techniques. Thus, it is important for a treating practitioner to record that the denial of benefits or the handling of benefits is having a negative impact on the health of her patient, either in a very direct fashion or simply by increasing stress and slowing down recovery. If the insurer's refusal to fund various treatment programs is having a negative impact on the patient's recovery, that should be noted as well. Also, if the patient is describing stress or concern arising out of the fact that they are being spied upon by private investigators hired by the insurer, this should be recorded in the physician's clinical notes and reporting as well. It is important that your doctor report the impact of the insurer's claims handling decisions/techniques on the insured. If the insurer knows that there is a third party monitoring the impact of their occasionally aggressive and abusive claims handling practices, they will be less likely to continue those practices against the patient.

CONCLUSION

While CFS/FM can be a devastating illness, it does not have to be an economic disaster for you and your family. Most employed individuals who become affected with the illness have access to at least one and often several sources of income replacement during the time they are unable to work while they are disabled. The key to minimizing the economic impact on you and your family is first to uncover all of the benefits you are entitled to while you are disabled. Then apply for the benefits promptly and effectively and aggressively pursue them until the government agency or responsible insurer relents and provides them to you in full. Insurers, in particular, may be reluctant to pay you benefits to which you are reasonably entitled, but if you pursue them with vigor, they will likely be forced to do the right thing in the end.

It is also important for you to assemble an effective team to advocate on your behalf at the earliest possible opportunity. There must be clear and effective communication between yourself, your family members, your financial advisors, and your medical practitioners in order to achieve quality results on your behalf. With properly qualified doctors commenting on your condition, honesty from yourself, and an experienced and aggressive lawyer advocating on your behalf, you will likely be successful.

CHAPTER SUMMARY

- CFS/FM can lead to significant economic strain. Due to the nature of the illnesses, patients are at a disadvantage when dealing with the often stressful claims processing.

- Insurers are often quick to dismiss CFS/FM claims.
- Utilizing legal assistance can be critical in securing appropriate benefits.
- Choose your lawyer wisely. Consider experience, knowledge, patience, and open communication.
- Honesty is always the best policy in dealing with lawyers. You should expect the same in return.
- The wheels of justice turn slowly. Do not expect a quick decision.
- Communicate well with your medical team in support of your case.
- Experienced, aggressive lawyers are challenging the dismissal of those who have devastating illnesses such as CFS/FM. This provides hope for all patients.

CHAPTER TEN

BUILDING YOUR TEAM AND BRINGING IT ALL TOGETHER

The road to recovery in CFS/FM includes building a team and support network. The most important provider in your health care team is your family doctor. While you may have to see other experts and specialists—including neurologists, rheumatologists, and gastroenterologists—ultimately your family doctor will be your lifeline. Your general practitioner should be considered your home base. In many states and provinces, you also have a choice of naturopathic doctors, who are licensed graduates of approved naturopathic colleges. They can provide guidance through the often murky waters of complementary and alternative medicine.

The purpose of the family practitioner is to provide you with the much-needed primary ongoing health care. Ideally, this person is a kind, caring, and informed individual who can give you supportive medical care throughout your illness. Unfortunately,

HERMAN®

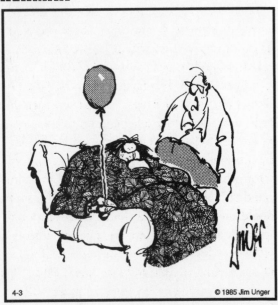

4-3   © 1985 Jim Unger

**"Mother, I thought we'd agreed –
'no luxuries.'"**

> **The Importance of the Doctor-Patient Relationship**
> - Two-thirds of CFS/FM patients are dissatisfied with the quality of their medical care.
> - Dissatisfied patients perceive doctors as dismissive, skeptical, or not knowledgeable about CFS/FM—advice given is inadequate or conflicting.
> - Satisfied patients perceive doctors as caring, supportive, and interested.
> - Patient evaluation is based less on ability to treat CFS/FM and more on interpersonal and informational skills.

not all doctors are well-informed regarding CFS/FM. If you do not feel supported by your primary care physician or even feel ridiculed because of your illness, I would not be entirely surprised. This, unfortunately, is a common tale that I hear from many of my patients. If at all possible, continue to look for a supportive practitioner. If this is not possible due to the lack of physicians in your area, continue to attend your family practitioner for ongoing supportive treatment; however, look for the ongoing emotional support needed to deal with a chronic illness elsewhere.

It is often helpful to go for ongoing supportive counseling, especially early on when the diagnosis is made. You need to deal with the loss of your job, your lifestyle, and your long-range goals. If your family doctor is not available to do this, look for counseling elsewhere, including psychotherapists, social workers, psychologists, ministers, etc. If these options are not available to you, look for other positive people who have the illness. These can be found through local support groups. The support group ideally should meet on a regular basis, be educational, have an agenda planned, and provide ongoing positive information. You should feel better after you attend the support group, not worse. If you walk out feeling terrible and a victim of your illness, do not go back. There are good and bad support groups. Make sure you find a good one.

SUPPORT GROUPS

If support groups are not available to you locally, there are ongoing provincial/state and federal support agencies. In Ontario, we have M.E. Ontario for Chronic Fatigue Syndrome and also Fibromyalgia Ontario. Federally, FM/ME Network Action is available in Canada. In the United States, there is the American Association of Chronic Fatigue Syndrome. Please see the Appendix for resources and Web sites available for information. If you do not have a computer, you can write to them. Most of the organizations have ongoing newsletters or journals.

FAMILY AND FINANCES

If you are in a long-term relationship, your spouse or partner is the most important person on your team. It is vitally important that the spouse is involved early on in your illness so that he or she has information about your illness and understands the long-term consequences of being chronically ill. Your partner will have to resume many of the duties that were previously shared in

HERMAN®

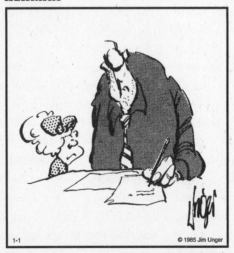

1-1   © 1985 Jim Unger

**"Mommy's not feeling too well, so I'm putting
you in charge of cooking and cleaning."**

your relationship. The degree of involvement obviously is determined by the degree of the fatigue/pain of the CFS/FM sufferer. If the patient is severely fatigued, the partner will have to assume responsibilities for cooking the meals, cleaning the house, caring for the children, transporting the children to their various activities, and also paying bills and long-term financial planning.

Because this is a long-term illness, it would be wise to immediately assess your finances once the diagnosis of CFS/FM has been made and to scale down your family's expenditures based on your reduced income if you have sick/disability benefits or no income at all if you won't be drawing disability benefits. Long-term financial planning may involve remortgaging the house to a lower, more manageable monthly payment. It may mean financial counseling at a credit-counseling center. Such centers help to look at the overall financial picture and to consolidate the debt into a lower monthly payment with a lower percentage interest. I have had a few patients who became so financially overloaded that they eventually had to declare bankruptcy due to the downturn in finances that resulted from their illness. For this reason, consider lawyers and financial advisors as potential team players.

If you have children, there can be no question that they will be affected by your illness. You as a parent will not be able to do all the things that you did in the past for them. Depending on the extent of your illness, you may have to grieve the loss of the ideal parenting role that you previously imagined—i.e., the always "doing" and "never say no" parent. This is not cause for despair; you will have to find new ways in which to share in your child's life. For example, one of my patients was totally bedridden for a while. During this time her husband brought their child to her bed, and she had about an hour of time with her each day, which she spent cuddling and talking quietly with her child. Another patient wanted to attend church with her children but was too severely fatigued to sit through an entire service. She spoke with her pastor ahead of time, and she arranged to have a special lawn chair brought in for her. She was able to lie down and listen to the service and feel that she was part of it.

In dealing with a chronic illness, you and your family need ongoing support. Your spouse and children are greatly involved with your illness. Many of the things that you used to do for them you cannot do now because you are too fatigued. This includes doing some or all of your household chores. Besides cleaning and cooking, it also includes things like driving kids to and from their appointments and participating in their social activities such as giving birthday parties. Your spouse can't do it all. He or she also needs help, so try to mobilize your parents, in-laws, neighbors, church, and friends to help sustain your spouse and your children.

If you have very little energy to walk, it might be helpful to look at getting a scooter so that you can stay as mobile as possible or a wheelchair if you have someone that can push you in it. For those of you with higher energy, I would suggest a walker with a seat. The walker will give you some stability while walking since your balance may often be off. Then if you need to have a rest, you can use the walker as a seat. Your family doctor can help you apply for these. If you are in the grocery store, lean on a shopping cart for added support while you walk.

MOBILITY

Regaining your mobility is vitally important. On your health care team you need to have a person who is familiar with rebuilding your muscle strength. This can be your family physician, a chiropractor, physiotherapist, osteopath, and/or massage therapist. What you need from this individual is someone who can help you to rebuild your muscle strength slowly and continuously. The more muscle you maintain and build, the higher your energy level will be. The difficulty is to try to improve your muscle strength without crashing.

The key to rebuilding strength is to have someone monitor your progress and also keep a record of it so that you know exactly what you are able to do on good and bad days. If you are totally bedridden, the range of motion exercises prescribed by a physiotherapist need to be done to keep your muscles mobile and functioning. As soon as possible you need to begin these exercises on your own to improve your muscle strength. You can do these exercises while you are in bed. I often recommend starting with only two to three repetitions of an exercise at a time. As you improve, you can add weight-bearing exercises that you should initially perform without weights. You start by doing the repetition using your own body weight for resistance. This helps to strengthen your muscles and tendons in preparation for eventually adding small weights. Once you are able to walk for approximately fifteen minutes, you can gradually build your muscles by adding small half-pound weights, for two or three repetitions. The weights should be increased very slowly according to exercise tolerance. Most normal people can start with eight repetitions, wait for a minute in between, and then repeat another eight repetitions of a particular muscle-strengthening exercise. It is always better to start with warm muscles, particularly after a physical activity such as walking. However, if you are too weak to walk, then your muscles will be warm if you are under covers before you get up in the morning or during a bath when you are sitting in warm water. *Strong Women Stay Young* by Miriam Nelson presents four upper body exercises and four lower body exercises. I again suggest starting with supervision with only three repetitions of the lower body exercises two times a week and three repetitions of the upper body exercises twice a week. So your exercise routine would be as follows: Monday: upper body; Tuesday: lower body; Wednesday: rest; Thursday: upper body; Friday: lower body. Your muscles need to rest the day after the exercises in order to repair and grow. If you do the muscle strengthening exercises every day you will actually damage your muscles. I find twice a week is the amount of muscle strengthening exercise that most patients can handle.

NUTRITIONAL FUEL

Your food is a key to your recovery, and a nutritionally oriented physician, naturopathic doctor, or nutritionist may have to guide you. You need to have nutritious meals throughout the day, beginning with breakfast. If you skip breakfast because you are too tired, you will continue to be too tired all day long. Begin eating within half an hour of getting up. If you are too tired to cook and you live alone, then you have to decide if you need help in the form of food brought in. An example of such a service would be Meals on Wheels. This service provides one dinner daily for a minimal fee. Alternatively, if you live alone you may benefit from cooking on your good days and freezing individual meals that you can reheat on your bad days. Frozen or canned entrées are also available. Bearing in mind the research from Dr. Logan's nutrition chapter, if at all possible try to find healthier frozen choices that have as few preservatives, such as MSG, as possible.

When energy levels are low in the morning, sometimes a liquid meal may be the way to go, and some patients get a boost from a smoothie. In a blender throw in a cup of milk or soy milk, 3 to 4 tablespoons of protein powder, such as proteins+, half a cup to a cup of blueberries or other fruit, and a tablespoon of oil such as flax or walnut. Blend it all up and enjoy. If you can't do this for yourself, consider a meal-replacement bar such as nutrilean+ and a glass of milk or dairy alternative such as soy or rice beverage. Some food is better than no food. Try to make it wholesome food if at all possible. Junk food really is junk for your immune system. Put food in your stomach within thirty minutes of getting up, even if you feel nauseated some mornings. You need fuel in your tank. And your body will thank you for it.

ADDITIONAL SUPPORT

Depending on your level of fatigue/pain, you may need either a bed bath in your home on an ongoing basis if you are bedridden or help to get you in and out of the bathtub if you are too fatigued to manage this on your own. My particular practice has a large number of very sick patients, so I know too well that some CFS/FM patients are at that level. Your family doctor may be helpful here in order to arrange an assessment by a visiting home-maker service to determine if you qualify for help with your bath on an ongoing basis. If this service is not available to you, try to mobilize family and friends to help you with your ongoing personal care. Sometimes hairdressers are available to visit in your home. Even if you can only manage this service occasionally, it helps to bolster your spirit to keep your hair looking neat and trimmed. Also try to boost your self-esteem by putting on a little makeup, such as lipstick or blush, each day. If you look in the mirror and you look better, you will also start to feel better about yourself.

If you can afford it, try to arrange for cleaning on a regular basis to keep the house running as smoothly as possible. If you have small children and your energy is very low, you will not be able to care for them. You will have to make arrangements for help either within or outside the home. Some of my patients have been able to enlist the help of their family and friends to do shifts to care for the children inside the home. Others have had the money to be able to hire full- or part-time nannies to care for their children. Because of their illness, some of my patients who are single mothers and live on the government disability pension qualify for government-supported daycare facilities for their children. These positions are difficult to access. There is often a long waiting list. Your doctor can help you with filling out forms to apply for this.

PREVENTION OF MCS

Try to reduce your exposure to chemicals in personal care products and cleaning products by using products that are as simple and odourless as possible. Since World War II, it has been estimated that there are about seventy thousand brand-new chemicals in our world. Yet our livers and kidneys, which we use to detoxify these chemicals, are still the same size. There is no "safe level" of exposure to chemicals. Try to use VOC-free paints in your home to reduce your chemical exposure. If you do need to renovate your home, try to do it in the summer months when all of your windows can be open and the chemicals can be blown outside with a fan. If you have to refinish wooden floors or cupboards with a veneer, remember that if you can still smell the finish you are inhaling it and it will remain inside your body until you can detoxify it. Canada Mortgage and Housing has a good Web site with resources to help guide you to less toxic products when renovating your home. Clean food, clean air, clean water, and clean environment—try to keep down your total body burden from chemical exposure.

YOU

As I mentioned early in the book, your CFS/FM recovery efforts require many coaches (such as doctors like myself) and team players (such as family and other CFS/FM patients), but the most important member of the team is you. Indeed, you are the key in building this team in an effort to support yourself. Your recovery process is an educational effort in how to maximize energy, while at the same time using it wisely to prevent setbacks. At the core of the recovery process is the need to learn how to continuously consider the importance of pacing. Of all the information contained in this book, the concept of pacing is perhaps the most important. After more than a decade of experience, my patients and I have come to realize that managing energy and pain through pacing will pay huge benefits.

You need to learn to feed yourself physically, emotionally, and spiritually. You need to learn how to manage your stress, your pain, and your ongoing sleep difficulties. You need to take control of the things that you can and live one day at a time. Start from where you are and build from there. Use the techniques that were introduced to you in previous chapters to help you control your stress, such as meditation, visualization, cognitive behav-

Summary of Healing Strategies in CFS/FM

1. Actively pace yourself. Essential to avoiding setbacks.
2. Improve sleep quality.
3. Improve pain management using individualized treatment.
4. Accept your illness. Work through denial, anger, depression, and other illness-related emotional responses.
5. Compare present health to illness onset, not your pre-illness state.
6. Eat healthy and nutritious foods. Remember healthy fats, complex carbohydrates, and fruits and vegetables. Reduce or eliminate caffeine, alcohol, and additives such as MSG and aspartame.
7. Take a multivitamin with adequate levels of minerals. This may require additional calcium and magnesium supplementation. Omega-3 fatty acids, Omega 6+, and probiotics may be useful.
8. Practice the techniques of mind-body medicine on a regular basis, particularly the relaxation response. Reduce the dominance of the sympathetic nervous system.
9. Appreciate your progress and accept and "forgive" yourself for setbacks.
10. Exercise, as tolerated, is important. Start with walking, then continue to strength training when you can walk twenty minutes.
11. With adequate energy, address unresolved emotional wounds.
12. Maintain optimism and have the intention that you will recover, and expect that recovery to be a gradual process.

ioral therapy, exercise, massage therapy, therapeutic touch, and prayer. Remain optimistic because there are some very intelligent scientists who are continuously searching for more clues to the CFS/FM puzzle. Practice energy conservation and harness the energy that you are giving up in wasted emotions such as anxiety and put it to use for your physical healing. This is accomplished by working through your feelings of denial, anger, depression, and anxiety so that you will have more available energy for physical healing.

A CFS/FM patient has one body with connected physical, emotional, and spiritual parts. Treat them all and listen to your body. It has a story to tell you. Stop being brain-driven and body-disconnected. Stop the crashing pattern that results from pushing your body to do more than it can manage. Stop writing checks with your brain that your body cannot cash. Be body- and brain-connected instead of disconnected. Integrate your parts into a whole being: this is mind-body medicine. You are a human being, not a human doing. You are more than the things you do for other people. Learn who you are and learn to be. You are a CFS/FM patient, yes, but you are one of a kind, and no one else will ever be you. Use this illness as an opportunity to discover the real you. Learn and grow from it. This sounds simple, but it is not easy. It is, in fact, often very difficult. The most challenging things in life are the things that make us stronger.

I hope that as you have read this book you have learned new tools to help you cope with your illness and have found inspiration to keep on trying as well as references for other sources of information about your illness.

Always remember that you are not alone. You are connected to so many people who have CFS/FM from all walks of life, and for all, there is reason to remain hopeful when travelling the bumpy road to recovery.

God bless you for taking the time to read this book.

Further Reading

Energy Conservation: Achieving a Balance of Work, Rest and Play. Carson, Gaya, Milantoni. Canadian Occupational Therapy Association, 700 Lawrence Avenue West, Suite 362, Toronto, Ontario M6A 3B4, Canada. 416-785-9230 or visit www.cota-health.ca.

The Fibromyalgia Cookbook. Shelly Ann Smith. Nashville: Cumberland House, 2002.

Managing Pain Before It Manages You. Margaret A. Caudill-Slosberg. New York: Guilford Press, 1994.

Fibromyalgia Aware magazine. Available at most bookstores and at www.fmaware.org.

CFS and FM clinical guidelines and more are available from The Haworth Press, 10 Alice Street, Binghamton, NY 13904. 800-429-6784, 607-771-0012, or visit www.haworthpress.com.

CFS/FM Organizations

The CFIDS Association of America
P.O. Box 220398
Charlotte, NC 28222-0398
704-365-2343
www.cfids.org

National ME/FM Action Network
3836 Carling Avenue
Nepean, ON K2K 2Y6
Canada
613-829-6667
www.mefmaction.net

National Chronic Fatigue Syndrome and Fibromyalgia Association
National Headquarters
P.O. Box 18426
Kansas City, MO 64133
816-313-2000
www.ncfsfs.org

The National CFIDS Foundation
103 Aletha Road
Needham, MA 02492
781-449-3535
Fax: 781-449–8606
www.ncf-net.org

The Myalgic Encephalomyelitis
Association of Ontario
P.O. Box 84522
2336 Bloor Street West
Toronto, Ontario, Canada
M6S 4Z7
416-222-8820
877-632-6682 (Ontario)
www.meao-cfs.on.ca

National Fibromyalgia Association
2200 Glassell Street, Suite "A"
Orange, CA 92865
714-921-0150
Fax: 714-921-6920
www.fmaware.org

Disability and Financial Aid

Social Security Administration
Office of Public Inquiries
Windsor Park Building
6401 Security Blvd.
Baltimore, MD 21235
800-772-1213
www.ssa.gov

Government of Canada
Income Security Department
800-277-9914 for Regional Office
www.hrsdc.gc.ca

Laboratory Testing for CFS

REDLABS U.S.A., Inc.
5625 Fox Avenue, Room 369
Reno, NV 89506
775-351-1890
Fax: 775-972-1300
www.REDLABSUSA.com

Legal Assistance

Association of Trial Lawyers of
America
The Leonard M. Ring Law Center
1050 31st Street, NW
Washington, DC 20007
800-424-2725 or 202-965-3500
www.atla.org

Ontario Trial Lawyers Association
4 Hughson Street South, Suite 301
Hamilton, ON L8N 3Z1
Canada
905-777-1777
Fax: 905-777-1667
www.otla.com

Complementary and Alternative Medicine

The American Association of
Naturopathic Physicians
3201 New Mexico Avenue, NW
Suite 350
Washington, DC 20016
866-538-2267 or 202-895-1392
Fax: 202-274-1992
www.naturopathic.org

American Holistic Medical
Association
12101 Menaul Boulevard, NE,
Suite C
Albuquerque, NM 87112
505-292-7788
Fax: 505-293-7582
www.holisticmedicine.org

Canadian Association of
Naturopathic Doctors
1255 Sheppard Avenue East,
Toronto
Canada M2K1E2
416-496-8633 or 800-551-4381
Fax: 416-496-8634
www.naturopathicassoc.ca

Mind-Body Medicine

Harvard Mind-Body Medical
Institute Programs
824 Boylston Street
Chestnut Hill, MA 02467
617-991-0102 or 866-509-0732
www.mbmi.org
Superb collection of instructional
tapes and CDs

**Environmental and Nutritional
Testing**

The Environmental Working Group
1436 U Street NW, Suite 100
Washington, DC 20009
202-667-6982
www.ewg.org
Provides up-to-date information
on mercury in fish and pesticides
on produce.

Nutrasource Diagnostics
Granbry Building, Suite 4
130 Research Lane
University of Guelph Research Park
Guelph, Ontario, Canada
N1G 5G3
877-557-7722
www.nutrasource.ca
Provides independent testing of
omega-3 fish oil supplements.

**Small Intestinal Bacterial
Overgrowth and Parasite Testing**

Integrative Care Centre of Toronto
3600 Ellesmere Road, Unit 4
Toronto, ON M1C 4Y8
www.thedoctors.ca

Nutritional Supplements

ehn inc
317 Adelaide Street West, 501
Toronto, ON M5V 1P9
416-977-8765 or 877-500-7888
Manufacturers of greens+, pro-
teins+, and the meal replacement
nutrilean+; also distribute the concentrated omega-3 EPA called
o3mega+ joy™
In the United States:
www.genuinehealth.com;
in Canada:
www.greenspluscanada.com.

Efamol Canada Inc.
35 Webster Street, Suite 103
Kentville, N.S., Canada, B4N 1H4
902-678-2727 or
888-318-5222
www.efamol.com

ZenBev™
Biosential Inc.
1543 Bayview Avenue, Suite 346
Toronto, ON M4G 3B5
Canada
800-735-4538 or 416-421-7445
www.zenbev.com

Probiotics

Yakult International (USA)
  3510 Torrance Boulevard,
  Suite 216
  Torrance, CA 90503
  310-792-1422
  Contact Hisashi Satoi at
  hsatoi@yakultusa.com
  www.yakult.co.jp/english/

Lactobacillus GG
  Culturelle™
  ConAgra Foods
  One ConAgra Drive
  Omaha, NE 68102
  402-595-4000 or 888-828-4242
  culturelle@conagrafoods.com
  Biodots for Meditation and Mind-
  Body Exercises

Stress Stop.com
  800-367-1604
  www.stressstop.com

Sauna

SaunaRay infrared saunas
  877-992-1100
  www.saunaray.com
  info@saunaray.com

Electrical Hypersensitivity

Less EMF Inc.
  141 Soller Heights Road
  Ghent, NY 12075
  518-672-6669
  www.lessemf.com

Institute for Building Biology
  Robert Steller, Director IBE
  Blue Mountain, Ontario, Canada
  519-599-1111
  www.buildingbiology.net
  buildingbiology@bellnet.ca

ABOUT THE AUTHORS

Alison Bested, a graduate of McMaster University Medical School, is a hematological pathologist who specializes in the complex medical problems related to chronic fatigue syndrome, fibromyalgia, and multiple chemical sensitivity. In addition to private practice, she teaches medical students and residents at the Environmental Health Clinic at the New Women's College Hospital and is a lecturer in the Department of Family and Community Medicine at the University of Toronto. She was chosen by Health Canada to participate in the writing of *Myalgic Encephalomyelitis/Chronic Fatigue Syndrome: Clinical Working Case Definition, Dignostic and Treatment Protocols.* She lives in Toronto, Ontario. **Alan C. Logan** is a faculty member of Harvard Medical School's Mind-Body Institute. He graduated magna cum laude from the State University of New York and was the valedictorian upon graduation from the Canadian College of Naturopathic Medicine in 2001. The nutrition editor of the *International Journal of Naturopathic Medicine* and a regular contributor to health magazines, Alan has been published in mainstream journals such as *Nutrition, Arthritis and Rheumatology, American Journal of Hypertension, Medical Hypotheses, Hospital Physician,* and *Medical Clinics of North America.* He lives in Westchester County, New York. **Russell Howe,** an attorney who specializes in medical disability cases, is currently president of the Ontario Trial Lawyer's Association. A significant number of his cases involve CFS/FM. He is a lecturer and has published articles on long-term disability. He lives in Aurora, Ontario.